# OPTIMUM
# NUTRITION
## FOR YOUR
# CHILD

## By the same author

# patrick HOLFORD
## & Deborah Colson

# OPTIMUM NUTRITION FOR YOUR CHILD

## HOW TO BOOST YOUR CHILD'S HEALTH, BEHAVIOUR AND IQ

piatkus

PIATKUS

First published in Great Britain in 2008 by Piatkus Books
Reprinted twice

This edition published 2010
Reprinted 2010

A CIP catalogue record for this book
is available from the British Library

ISBN 978-0-7499-5353-9

Typeset in Monotype Dante by Phoenix Photosetting, Chatham, Kent
www.phoenixphotosetting.co.uk
Printed and bound by CPI Mackays, Chatham ME5 8TD

Papers used by Piatkus are natural, renewable and recyclable
products sourced from well-managed forests and certified
in accordance with the rules of the Forest Stewardship Council.

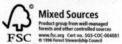

**Mixed Sources**
Product group from well-managed
forests and other controlled sources
www.fsc.org  Cert no. SGS-COC-004081
© 1996 Forest Stewardship Council
FSC

Piatkus
An imprint of
Little, Brown Book Group
100 Victoria Embankment
London EC4Y 0DY

An Hachette UK Company
www.hachette.co.uk

www.piatkus.co.uk

# Contents

# Acknowledgements

We'd like to thank the many scientists whose research we have referred to, who have tirelessly put the role of optimum nutrition for children's development on the map, often funding their own research. Special thanks go to our editors Jillian, Tiara and Lisa at Piatkus/Littlebrown for their invaluable contribution. But, most of all, we'd like to thank the many children and their parents with whom we've worked at the Brain Bio Centre and Food for the Brain – it is they who have taught us the most.

---

**Abbreviations and measures**

1 gram (g) = 1,000 milligrams (mg) = 1,000,000 micrograms (mcg, also written μg).

All vitamins are measured in milligrams or micrograms. Vitamins A, D and E used to be measured in International Units (ius), a measurement designed to standardise the various forms of these vitamins that have different potencies.

6mcg of beta-carotene, the vegetable precursor of vitamin A, is, on average, converted into 1mcg of retinol, the animal form of vitamin A. So, 6mcg of beta-carotene is called 1mcgRE (RE stands for retinol equivalent). Throughout this book beta-carotene is referred to in mcgRE.

1mcg of retinol (mcgRE) = 3.3ius of vitamin A
1mcgRE of beta-carotene = 6mcg of beta-carotene
100ius of vitamin D = 2.5mcg
100ius of vitamin E = 67mg
1 pound (lb) = 16 ounces (oz)     2.2lbs = 1 kilogram (kg)
1 pint = 0.6 litres               1.76 pints = 1 litre
In this book calories means kilocalories (kcals)

### References and further sources of information

Hundreds of references from respected scientific literature have been used in the writing of this book. Details of specific studies referred to are listed on pages 279–90. Other supporting research for statements made is available from the library at the Institute for Optimum Nutrition (ION) (see page 292). ION also offers information services, including literature search and library search facilities, for those readers who want to access scientific literature on specific subjects. On page 291 you will find a list of the best books to read to enable you to dig deeper in to the topics covered. You will find many of the topics touched on in this book covered in detail in Patrick's feature articles, available at www.patrick holford.com. If you want to stay up to date with all that is new and exciting in this field we recommend you subscribe to Patrick's *100% Health* newsletter, details of which are on the website.

# Our Work With Children

Probably the single most important thing you can do for your child's future health and happiness is to give them optimum nutrition. Ever since the 1980s when we researched the IQ boosting effects of giving children multivitamins, we have continued to explore what 'optimum' really means. I (Patrick) run the Food for the Brain Foundation, an educational charity that exists to help raise awareness about the importance of nutrition for maximising you and your child's potential. Have a look at our website www.foodforthebrain.org. I (Deborah) trained at the Institute for Optimum Nutrition, and specialise in helping children with special educational needs from ADHD to autism at the Brain Bio Centre in Richmond.

Together, we work with individual children and with schools and care homes to help them deliver optimum nutrition to all children. This 'hands on' work has really helped us find out both what works for children and what's practical for parents and carers.

The results of our Food for the Brain schools projects have been remarkable. Through simply changes in diet, plus daily nutritional supplements, we have helped under-performing children, and those with special educational needs make big improvements.

For example, in one school, Cricket Green, parents rated a 15 per cent reduction in defiance and oppositional behaviour, an 18 per cent reduction in anxiousness and shyness and a 25 per cent reduction in psychosomatic symptoms such as tummy aches and headaches etc. The head teacher, Celia Dawson, reported three clear changes: 'improvements in the quality of communication and use of language, greater attention to tasks and therefore improved quality in work such as handwriting, and parents reporting changes in mood swings with pupils being calmer.'

In another, a poorly performing primary school, SAT scores went up by 21 per cent in Maths, 15 per cent in English and 14 per cent in Science. 'We are really delighted with these results,' said the school head Gwen Clifford. 'The Food for the Brain project has had a very positive impact in school.'

But what really counts is the transformation of the children. 'Her reading, writing and confidence have improved incredibly,' said one mum. 'Her mood is so much better. She's much more communicative,' said another. 'He used to be aggressive. Now he's much calmer and even says sorry when he loses his temper. This never happened before,' said a mum of a child with ADHD. 'He's gone to the top of the class. He's focusing much better, thinking more clearly and is generally happier and healthier.'

We hope that by applying what you learn in this book, your child will be healthier and happier and maximise their potential in school and in life. That, we believe, is the greatest legacy any parent can give their child.

# Introduction

We all want our children to be healthy and happy, intelligent and resourceful, and to have the full range of life skills they will need to live productively and well.

We give them as much love and attention as we can to enable them to develop physically, mentally and emotionally. We teach them how to walk and talk. We read books about parenting and we try not to make the same mistakes our parents made. We engage and stimulate our children, we show them how to get the most out of what they're learning at school, and we support them through the challenging process of becoming an adult.

But in all of this do we really take into account the fact that every step a child takes – whether it's their first toddle on the kitchen floor or their first teenage relationship – depends on how well their body is working? And that, in turn, depends to a large extent on how well their body is nourished?

We have more than 20 years' experience of working with children and in this book we're going to show you, step by step, what optimum nutrition really means for your child, whether they are one or 15.

## How to use this book

**In Part 1 – Food and Your Child**, you'll discover why the right food is so important for your child's health and development, and you'll learn what to feed your child – and what to avoid.

**In Part 2 – Give Your Child a Head Start**, we describe the foods and supplements that will boost your child's educational performance and potential for happiness by improving their mood and behaviour, sharpening their memory and concentration, and raising their IQ.

**In Part 3 – Solving Problems**, we give you nutritional solutions to maximise your child's physical and emotional health, as well as improve specific conditions such as asthma, insomnia, obesity, autism and frequent infections.

**In Part 4 – Making it Real**, we demonstrate how to put all this knowledge into action and explain what to do to feed your child properly, from infancy to teenage years. You'll find plenty of practical tips, as well as advice on choosing the right supplements.

The biggest gift we can give our children is a good start on the road to a long and healthy life. A huge part of that is making the best nutrition available to them, to help them feel alert, energetic, happy and disease-free, with a clear mind and a focused intelligence. This book is written with that goal in mind.

Wishing you and your children the best of health,

*Patrick Holford and Deborah Colson*

## PART 1

·

# FOOD AND YOUR CHILD

In a very literal sense your child is made of food, so what they eat has a direct effect on how they feel and function. In this part of the book you'll find out why optimum nutrition is important for your child and what you should – and shouldn't – feed them.

# Chapter 1

# What little boys and girls are made of

Have you ever wondered what a newborn baby's skin, bones, blood, flesh, organs and so on are made of? Well it's certainly not puppy dogs' tails and it isn't sugar and spice either! You'll be aware that bones are made from calcium, amongst other things, and that blood contains iron. You may also know that flesh is made up of protein and that more than half of a baby's brain is constructed from a special type of fat called an essential fat. But where do the calcium, iron, protein and essential fat – not to mention the 50 other essential nutrients that make up a baby – come from? The answer is food. From the moment of conception to the arrival, nine months later, of a fully functioning, living, breathing human being, a baby is using the food that it receives in the womb to grow and develop.

And that's just the beginning of the story. A newborn baby grows at a fantastic rate, tripling its birth weight in the first year. This growth is only possible because the particles of food that he or she is eating are used, literally, to build a bigger baby. Adults have a constant need for nutrients, too, to maintain and repair their bodies. For instance, we renew our skin every 20 days and the lining of our gut every four days. However, unlike adults, children's bodies not only undergo this constant maintenance and repair, but they are also growing and developing at the same time, so it's even more important that they get plenty of the right nutrients.

What this means is that your child should consume the right carbohydrates, fats and proteins, the three major nutrients – or macronutrients – that are used to build and fuel your child, as well as the many vital vitamins and minerals – or micronutrients – that are essential for keeping their body running smoothly. However, food also contains anti-nutrients, which are substances such as refined sugar, damaged fats, chemical food additives and toxic minerals that can disrupt the good work of the nutrients, so you should steer your child clear of these.

We do understand, though, that knowing what a child should be eating is one thing and actually getting them to eat it is quite another. Left to their own devices, children will naturally narrow the range of foods that they like until they'll only eat three things, one of which will be chips! It can be very frustrating at times, but one of your jobs as a parent is to continually counteract this tendency, and to broaden the range of foods they consume.

Of course, everybody knows that it's important to feed a child a healthy diet and yet in the UK one third of children are overweight or obese, and there are three children with asthma in the average classroom. According to the latest figures from the Office for National Statistics, one in ten children aged five to 16 has a clinically recognisable mental disorder, such as anxiety, depression, hyperactivity or autism. What's more, incidences of 'lifestyle diseases' such as type II diabetes and fatty liver disease, previously only seen in overweight and unhealthy older adults, are now appearing in children in increasing numbers. In fact, the current generation of young people is the first that can expect to live shorter lives than their parents. However, if you're reading this book you've already taken the first step towards ensuring that your child doesn't become one of these shocking statistics and you obviously want to set your child up for optimum health for life.

## Chapter 2

·

# Not all carbohydrates are created equal

**W**hile a cat likes the taste of protein, humans are principally attracted to the taste of sweet things. This inherent attraction towards sweetness worked well for early man, because most things in nature that are sweet aren't poisonous and are safe to eat. It worked well for plants, too. They hid their seeds in their fruit, waiting for people to pass by, eat the fruit and deposit the seed some distance from the original plant, along with an 'organic manure' starter kit!

In fact, fruit and other plant matter consist mainly of carbohydrate and the sweetness that people are attracted to is actually the carbohydrate. This is because, although it's possible for us to use protein and fat for energy, carbohydrate is what the human body is designed to run on.

Carbohydrates should make up a quarter to one third of each of your child's meals. When your child eats complex carbohydrates like wholegrains, vegetables, beans or lentils, or simpler carbohydrates such as fruit, the body does exactly what it is designed to do: it digests these foods and gradually releases their potential energy. What's more, all the nutrients that the body needs for digestion and metabolism are present in those wholefoods, and they also contain fibre, a less-digestible type of carbohydrate, which helps keep the digestive system running smoothly.

However, man has discovered how to take the carbohydrate from plants, extract the sweetness and leave the rest, which is very bad news for our nutrition. All forms of concentrated sugar – white sugar, brown sugar, malt, glucose, honey and syrup – release sugar into the blood quickly, causing a rapid increase in blood sugar levels. If this sugar isn't required by the body it's put into storage, eventually emerging as fat. Unlike natural sources of sweetness and carbohydrate, such as fruit, most concentrated forms of sugar are also devoid of vitamins and minerals. White sugar, for example, has around 90 per cent of its vitamins and minerals removed. Without vitamins and minerals our metabolism becomes inefficient, contributing to low energy levels and mood, and poor weight control.

## How plants make carbohydrates

Plants make carbohydrates by using energy from the sun, which they absorb through their leaves, to combine carbon and oxygen from the air with hydrogen and more oxygen from the water they take in through their roots. This process is called photosynthesis.

Your child eats the carbohydrate and, in the presence of oxygen from the air, their body breaks it down, releasing the stored solar energy that then provides energy for their body and mind.

## Sweet and simple

Fruit contains a simple sugar called fructose, which needs no digesting and can therefore enter the bloodstream quickly, like the simple sugars glucose, which is found in starchy foods, or sucrose, which is the sugar we might put in tea. However, unlike them it is classified as slow-releasing. This is because cells only run on glucose and the body can't use fructose as it is. As a result, the body has to convert the fructose into glucose, which effectively slows down the fructose's effect on the metabolism. Lactose, the sugar in milk, works in a similar way, because it's made up of a type of glucose and something called galactose. The glucose is fast-releasing, while the galactose is slow-releasing.

Some fruits, such as grapes and dates, also contain pure glucose and are therefore fairly fast-releasing. Apples, on the other hand, contain mainly fructose and so are slow-releasing, while bananas contain both and therefore raise blood sugar levels quite speedily. All fresh fruit, however, whether it's fast- or slow-releasing, has two big advantages. One is fibre, which slows down the release of the sugars contained in the fruit. The other is vitamins, which are essential for making full use of the carbohydrates (see chapter 5 for more on this).

What about dried fruit? In a nutshell, it's problematic. This is because, weight for weight, it obviously contains much less water than fresh fruit, and this both concentrates the sugar and makes it less filling, so you can end up packing away quite a lot of it without realising. Moreover, the fibre in dried apples, for instance, is less effective at slowing down sugar release. Dried fruit is a good alternative to sweets, but don't make it a substitute for fresh and when you do give it to your kids, soak it first, so they won't eat as much of it.

Refined carbohydrates such as white bread, white rice and refined cereals have a similar effect to refined sugar, while oats are more 'complex', which slows down their release of sugar. The process of refining or even cooking starts to break down complex carbohydrates into simple carbohydrates called malt (officially maltose), in effect predigesting them. When your child eats simple carbohydrates he or she gets a rapid increase in blood sugar levels and a corresponding surge in energy, which you will have seen if you have ever picked your child up from a birthday party and opened the door on a roomful of kids bouncing off the walls! The surge, however, is followed by a drop as the body scrambles to balance the blood sugar levels and overshoots. This drop in blood sugar level will manifest in your child as the whines and grizzles, irritability and tantrums that typically follow the birthday party sugar rush.

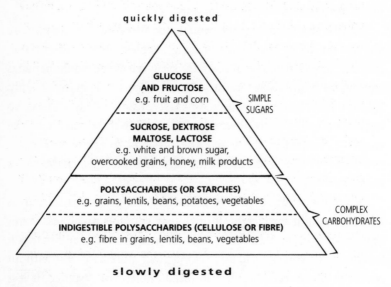

*The sugar family*

As we've said, carbohydrates are an important source of fuel for your child. The trick is to keep the supply even. Too much and you get the wall-bouncing effect. Too little and your child could experience symptoms such as fatigue, irritability, dizziness, insomnia, aggression, anxiety, sweating (especially at night), poor concentration, excessive thirst, depression, crying spells or blurred vision. So for your child to be able to think with clarity, behave rationally and have steady energy levels, it's vital that their glucose supply stays steady and even.

CASE HISTORY *John, age 4*

John's parents brought him to see us at the Brain Bio Centre in London because they were concerned about his severe speech and language delay, and his inability to concentrate. We screened him for various biochemical imbalances and analysed his diet. While fairly typical for a four-year-old and not especially unhealthy, the food John ate contained a lot of hidden sugar, so we recommended that his parents reduce all sources of sugar, including bananas (they contain fast-releasing sugar). According to his parents, child minder and teachers, within a few short weeks John was a different child. His scribblings turned into drawings which he could talk about. He slept better at night and no longer needed to nap during the day. He was much calmer, his comprehension improved and he began trying to do jigsaw puzzles. However, one day during this period John's granddad gave him half a banana, thinking it was allowed on the 'diet' and the effect was incredible. 'He went completely beserk,' John's mother told us, 'and ran from one end of the house to the other for an hour until the effect of the banana wore off.' Not surprisingly, having seen just how sensitive John is to it, his doting grandparents won't be giving him any sneaky sugar again!

## The ups and downs of blood sugar

When your child consumes a lot of fast-releasing carbohydrate all at once – say, a fizzy drink and biscuits or white toast and jam – their blood sugar levels will soar. Glucose is powerful stuff, and can actually damage nerves and blood vessels. The body copes with this by enlisting the help of the hormone insulin, which is released from the pancreas when a burst of glucose hits your child's bloodstream.

Once in the blood, insulin escorts the glucose into cells, where it's used for energy. Any excess – and if your child has overdosed on refined carbohydrates there's bound to be some – is stored, in a form called glycogen, in other parts of the body, such as the muscles and liver. When these stores are full, any remaining glucose is converted to body fat. A diet high in sugar is probably the biggest cause of obesity or overweight in children (see chapter 12 for more on this).

In the 'sugar overdose' scenario – after a big bowl of processed, sweetened cereal, say, or a bag of sweets at the cinema – the body responds to what it sees as a dangerous situation by releasing more insulin than normal. As a result, too much glucose can actually be escorted out of the bloodstream. This leaves your child with a blood sugar level that's too low and they experience a subsequent crash in energy. We've seen how nasty the symptoms of low blood sugar can be, but, even worse, your child is then likely to crave more of what caused the problem in the first place – sugar – just to get rid of the unpleasant feelings, and round we go again. It's a vicious cycle that leads to more cravings, more extreme mood fluctuations, and progressively poorer concentration, behaviour and energy levels.

## BLOOD SUGAR CHECK

Check your child's blood sugar balance by answering the questions below:

Does your child...

- [ ] usually eat white bread, rice or pasta instead of brown or wholegrain?
- [ ] crave sugar, sweets or refined carbohydrates such as chocolate, biscuits, toast and jam or sweetened cereals?
- [ ] have sugary foods or drinks at regular intervals during the day?
- [ ] crave caffeinated drinks such as colas?

☐ sometimes skip meals, especially breakfast?

☐ seem to be slow to get going in the morning?

☐ have energy slumps during the day?

☐ sometimes lose concentration or have a poor attention span?

☐ get dizzy, dopey or irritable if they don't eat often?

☐ seem to lack energy?

*If you answer 'yes' to five or more of these questions, the chances are your child's blood sugar balance is less than perfect.*

## Sugar imbalance and your child

Seesawing blood sugar levels can also affect children's IQ – and not in a good way! Research at the Massachusetts Institute of Technology in the US found a massive 25 per cent difference between the IQ scores of children who were in the top fifth of the population for consumption of sugar and other refined carbohydrates, compared with children who were in the bottom fifth.[1] So staying away from white bread, processed cereals and sugar seems to be crucial to having a higher IQ.

But that's not all. To maximise mental performance your child needs to have that all-important even supply of glucose to the brain. This has been well proven by Professor David Benton at Swansea University, who has found that dips in blood glucose are directly associated with poor attention, poor memory and aggressive behaviour.[2] Sugar has been implicated in aggressive behaviour,[3-4] anxiety,[5-6] hyperactivity and attention deficit,[7] depression,[8] eating disorders,[9] fatigue[10] and learning difficulties.[11-12]

Moreover, dietary studies consistently reveal that hyperactive children eat more sugar than other children,[13] and that reducing dietary sugar halves the need for disciplinary interventions among young offenders.[14] A study of 265 hyperactive children found that more than three-quarters displayed an abnormal balance in their glucose levels.[15]

It's not just the effects on children's mental and emotional health that are worrying, either. As we've mentioned, sugar-related diseases such as obesity and diabetes are also on the increase in children. Diabetes is an extreme form of blood sugar imbalance. This condition arises when the body can no longer produce sufficient insulin to adequately manage blood sugar levels. The result is too much glucose in the blood and not enough for the cells. One of the tell-tale signs is a continuous raging thirst as the body tries to dilute the excess blood sugar by stimulating us to drink. Excess sugar in the blood can damage blood vessels and nerves, which is why diabetes is the primary cause of blindness and limb amputations in adults.

Type 1 diabetes, which used to be called child-onset diabetes, usually develops in early childhood and is recognised as an auto-immune condition, because the body's immune system attacks its insulin-producing cells. Children with this medical condition produce no, or very little, insulin and will need to inject insulin after meals every day, probably for life. Children with type 1 diabetes will benefit from eating to keep their blood sugar balanced, because the fluctuations in their blood sugar levels will be less extreme, requiring lower levels of injected insulin, and they will experience fewer episodes of high or low blood sugar and the health risks these bring.

Type II diabetes is by far the more prevalent form of this disease and the incidence is growing rapidly. Type II diabetes used to be known as adult-onset diabetes, because it was only found in older adults. It's a 'lifestyle' disease in that it's the result of making unhealthy lifestyle choices and consuming excess sugar, not taking enough exercise and being overweight. People with this condition may still be producing some insulin, but they may have become resistant to its effect. Sadly, we are seeing more and more cases of teenagers, and even younger children, being diagnosed with this condition. Most people with type II diabetes can manage their blood sugar levels adequately by simply eating to keep their blood sugar balanced, although some may require medication.

Similarly, fatty liver or *hepatic steatosis*, a disease of the liver, was virtually unheard of in children a generation ago, yet is now seen increasingly in overweight children. The prevailing view was that excess fat in the diet leads to excess fat accumulating in the liver. However, recent research suggests that it may have more to do with sugar than fat. A study on mice carried out at the Children's Hospital Boston in the US gave mice diets that contained the same number of calories, but which consisted of either fast- or slow-releasing carbohydrates. After six months the mice all weighed the same, but there were real differences in the composition of their bodies. The mice that had eaten the slow-releasing carbs were lean, with normal amounts of fat throughout their bodies, whereas the mice on the fast-releasing carbs had twice the amount of fat in their bodies, blood and livers.[16] Interestingly, the French delicacy foie gras – the fatty liver of a duck or goose – is produced by over-feeding the animals with grains that contain fast-releasing carbo-hydrates. A clinical trial is now underway at the Children's Hospital Boston to gauge if a low-sugar diet can reverse fatty liver disease in overweight children.

## The carbs that keep blood sugar even

Now that we know how important the release rate of carbohydrates is, how can you tell which foods are fast-releasing and which are slow-releasing? As a general rule, you can assume that whole, unprocessed foods are the slowest to release their sugar. Beyond this, you can use a measure called the glycemic load (GL).

In essence, GL measures the effect of a food on the levels of glucose in the blood. Foods with a GL of less than ten are good and should be the staple foods of your child's diet. Foods with a GL of 11 to 14 are OK and can be eaten in moderation. Foods with a GL higher than 15 should be avoided. Beware of combining two moderate-GL foods in one meal, though, because when they're eaten together their GL adds up to a high combined GL. For example, a crumpet, which has a moderate GL, eaten with unsweetened peanut butter, which has a low GL, remains moderate, while the GL score of a crumpet with a teaspoon of honey, which also has a moderate GL, shoots up.

If you're already familiar with something called the glycemic index (GI), you can think of GL as 'the new improved' GI. Put simply, GI tells you how fast or slow the sugar in a food is released, whereas GL tells you not only the speed of release of the sugar, but also how much of the sugar there is in the food. In other words, GI tells you nothing about quantity. The GI of a sack of potatoes is the same as the GI of a single potato, whereas GL relates to the serving size, so you know what sort of sugar effect you're getting for a serving of a particular food. A good example of where GL is more helpful than GI is watermelon. Watermelon has a high GI, because it contains fast-releasing sugar, but watermelon contains so little of this sugar that eating a medium slice has little effect on blood sugar levels, so it consequently has a low GL.

The chart opposite gives the GL score of an average serving of a range of common foods. You can start to use this now by checking out what your child eats for breakfast. If they start the day with puffed rice cereal and raisins, both of which have a high GL score, they're getting rocket fuel first thing in the morning – and that means that a couple of hours later their blood glucose and energy will plummet. But give them oat flakes, sweetened with a chopped apple, both of which are slow-releasing, and their energy and concentration will last right through to lunch.

## GLYCEMIC LOAD OF COMMON FOODS

| Food | GL per serving | Serving size in g | Looks like |
|---|---|---|---|
| **Bakery products** | | | |
| Muffin – low carb | 5 | – | 1 muffin |
| Apple and almond cake | 5 | – | 1 medium slice |
| Carrot and walnut cake | 5 | – | 1 medium slice |
| Muffin – apple, made without sugar | 9 | 60 | 1 muffin |
| Muffin – apple, made with sugar | 13 | 60 | 1 muffin |
| Crumpet | 13 | 50 | 1 crumpet |
| Muffin – apple, oat, sultana, made from packet mix | 14 | 50 | 1 muffin |
| Muffin – bran | 15 | 57 | 1 muffin |
| Banana cake, made without sugar | 16 | 80 | 1 medium slice |
| Muffin – blueberry | 17 | 57 | 1 muffin |
| Muffin – banana, oat and honey | 17 | 50 | 1 muffin |
| Croissant | 17 | 57 | 1 croissant |
| Doughnut | 17 | 47 | 1 plain doughnut |
| Sponge cake, plain | 17 | 63 | 1 slice |
| Muffin – carrot | 20 | 57 | 1 muffin |
| **Breads** | | | |
| Volkenbrot wholemeal rye bread | 5 | 20 | 1 slice |
| Rice bread, high-amylose | 5 | 20 | 1 small slice |
| Rice bread, low-amylose | 5 | 20 | 1 small slice |
| Wholemeal rye bread | 5 | 20 | 1 thin slice |
| Wheat tortilla (Mexican) | 5 | 30 | 1 tortilla |
| Chapatti, white wheat flour, thin, with green gram | 5 | 30 | 1 chapatti |
| Rye kernel (pumpernickel) bread | 6 | 30 | 1 slice |
| Sourdough rye bread | 6 | 30 | 1 slice |
| White, high-fibre bread | 9 | 30 | 1 thick slice |
| Wholemeal (wholewheat) wheat flour bread | 9 | 30 | 1 thick slice |
| Gluten-free fibre-enriched bread | 9 | 30 | 1 thick slice |
| Gluten-free multigrain bread | 10 | 30 | 1 slice |
| Light rye bread | 10 | 30 | 1 slice |

continues →

| Food | GL per serving | Serving size in g | Looks like |
| --- | --- | --- | --- |
| White wheat flour bread | 10 | 30 | 1 slice |
| Pitta bread, white | 10 | 30 | 1 pitta |
| Wheat flour flatbread | 10 | 30 | 1 slice |
| Gluten-free white bread | 11 | 30 | 1 slice |
| Corn tortilla | 12 | 50 | 1 tortilla |
| Middle Eastern flatbread | 15 | 30 | 1 slice |
| Baguette, white, plain | 15 | 30 | ¹/₁₃ baton |
| Bagel, white, frozen | 25 | 70 | 1 bagel |
| **Crispbreads and crackers** | | | |
| Rough Oat Cakes™ (Nairn's) | 2 | 10 | 1 oat cake |
| Fine Oat Cakes™ (Nairn's) | 3 | 9 | 1 oat cake |
| Cheesey Oat Cakes™ (Nairn's) | 3 | 8 | 1 oat cake |
| Cream cracker | 11 | 25 | 2 biscuits |
| Rye crispbread | 11 | 25 | 2 biscuits |
| Water cracker | 17 | 25 | 3 biscuits |
| Puffed rice cakes | 17 | 25 | 3 biscuits |
| **Dairy products and alternatives** | | | |
| Plain yoghurt, no sugar | 3 | 200 | 1 small pot |
| Non-fat yoghurt, plain, no sugar | 3 | 200 | 1 small pot |
| Soya yoghurt (Provamel) | 7 | 200 | 1 large bowl |
| Soya milk, no sugar | 7 | (250ml) | 1 glass |
| Low-fat yoghurt, fruit, sugar (Ski) | 7.5 | 150 | 1 small pot |
| **Fruit and fruit products** | | | |
| Blackberries | 1 | 120 | 1 medium bowl |
| Blueberries | 1 | 120 | 1 medium bowl |
| Raspberries | 1 | 120 | 1 medium bowl |
| Strawberries, fresh, raw | 1 | 120 | 1 medium bowl |
| Cherries, raw | 3 | 120 | 1 medium bowl |
| Grapefruit, raw | 3 | 120 | ½ medium |
| Pear, raw | 4 | 120 | 1 medium |
| Melon/cantaloupe, raw | 4 | 120 | ½ small |
| Watermelon, raw | 4 | 120 | 1 medium slice |
| Peaches, raw or canned in natural juice | 5 | 120 | 1 |

continues →

| Food | GL per serving | Serving size in g | Looks like |
|---|---|---|---|
| Apricots, raw | 5 | 120 | 4 apricots |
| Oranges, raw | 5 | 120 | 1 large |
| Plum, raw | 5 | 120 | 4 |
| Apples, raw | 6 | 120 | 1 small |
| Kiwi fruit, raw | 6 | 120 | 1 |
| Pineapple, raw | 7 | 120 | 1 medium slice |
| Grapes, raw | 8 | 120 | 16 |
| Mango, raw | 8 | 120 | 1½ slices |
| Apricots, dried | 9 | 60 | 6 apricots |
| Fruit cocktail, canned (Del Monte) | 9 | 120 | Small tin |
| Papaya, raw | 10 | 120 | Half a small papaya |
| Prunes, pitted | 10 | 60 | 6 prunes |
| Apple, dried | 10 | 60 | 6 rings |
| Banana, raw | 12 | 120 | 1 small |
| Apricots, canned in light syrup | 12 | 120 | 1 small tin |
| Lychees, canned in syrup and drained | 16 | 120 | 1 small tin |
| Figs, dried, tenderised (Dessert Maid) | 16 | 60 | 3 |
| Sultanas | 25 | 60 | 30 |
| Raisins | 28 | 60 | 30 |
| Dates, dried | 42 | 60 | 8 |
| **Jams and spreads** | | | |
| Pumpkin seed butter | 1 | 16 | 1 tbsp |
| Peanut butter, no sugar | 1 | 16 | 1 tbsp |
| Blueberry spread, no sugar | 1 | 10 | 1 dessertspoon |
| Apricot fruit spread, reduced sugar | 2 | 10 | 1 dessertspoon |
| Orange marmalade | 3 | 10 | 1 dessertspoon |
| Strawberry jam | 3 | 10 | 1 dessertspoon |
| **Savoury snack foods** | | | |
| Eggs – boiled | 0 | – | 2 medium |
| Cottage cheese | 2 | 120 | ½ medium tub |
| Egg mayonnaise | 2 | 120 | ½ medium tub |
| Hummus | 6 | 200 | 1 small tub |
| Olives, in brine | 1 | 50 | 7 |

continues →

| Food | GL per serving | Serving size in g | Looks like |
|---|---|---|---|
| Peanuts | 1 | 50 | 2 medium handfuls |
| Cashew nuts, salted | 3 | 50 | 2 medium handfuls |
| Potato crisps, plain, salted | 7 | 30 | 1 small packet |
| Popcorn, salted | 10 | 25 | 1 small packet |
| Pretzels, oven-baked, traditional wheat flavour | 16 | 30 | 15 |
| Corn chips, plain, salted | 17 | 50 | 18 |
| **Sweet snack foods** | | | |
| GoodCarb™ Real Belgian Chocolate Brownie (all three flavours) | 3 | 45 | 1 bar |
| Fruitus apple cereal bar | 5 | 35 | 1 |
| Euroviva Rebar fruit and veg bar | 8 | 50 | 1 |
| Apricot fruit bar (dried apricot filling in wholemeal pastry) | 12 | 35 | 1 |
| Muesli bar with dried fruit | 13 | 30 | 1 |
| Chocolate bar, milk, plain (Mars/Cadbury/Nestlé) | 14 | 50 | 1 |
| Twix® biscuit and caramel bar (Mars) | 17 | 60 | 1 bar (2 fingers) |
| Snickers® bar (Mars) | 19 | 60 | 1 |
| Polos peppermint sweets (Nestlé) | 21 | 30 | 16 |
| Jelly beans, assorted colours | 22 | 30 | 9 |
| Kellogg's Pop-Tarts™, double choc | 24 | 50 | 1 |
| Mars Bar® | 26 | 60 | 1 |

*A comprehensive list of the GL of foods is available in* The Optimum Nutrition Bible *and* The Low-GL Diet Bible *or online at www.holforddiet.com.*

# How to keep your child in perfect balance

As is abundantly clear from the chart above, the GL of some foods is through the roof and bound to play havoc with your child's blood sugar balance. You may have had a few shocks – baguettes and bagels have quite a high GL, for instance – but, as you'll discover, it's amazingly easy to find delicious and thoroughly satisfying substitutes. Here are a few examples of what your child should, and should not, be eating to keep his or her blood glucose level in good balance:

| Instead of... | Eat |
| --- | --- |
| White toast and jam | Wholegrain toast and baked beans |
| Cornflakes | Porridge with raspberries |
| Croissants and baguettes | Wholegrain rye breads |
| White rice | Wholemeal spaghetti |
| Chocolate bars | Raw vegetable crudités |
| Bananas | Berries, apples or oranges |
| Crackers or rice cakes | Oatcakes |

We'll look at how to do this in more detail later on, but now let's look at what should be on your child's plate – and what needs to stay on the supermarket shelves.

## Sugar – the long goodbye

Weaning your child off sugar is a big part of the switch to eating for blood sugar balance. For both you and your child, the easiest way to do this is to decrease the sugar content of your child's diet slowly and gradually over time, so that they will get used to less sweetness without noticing it too much.

The first thing to do is swap the obvious sources of sugar, such as sweets, biscuits and puddings, for lower sugar alternatives. Make it easy on yourself and empty the cupboards of the sugar-laden rubbish. It's a lot easier to say to your child, 'There isn't any of that' than to say 'No, you can't have that.' If you're a sugar junkie, you'll need work on your own sugar withdrawal, too!

While we don't advocate that your child eats dried fruit in place of fresh fruit, it does make a good substitute for occasional sweets.

Oat flapjacks are a good replacement for biscuits, because the oats have a lower GL than refined wheat flour. Of course, an apple would be even better as a snack. As with sweets and biscuits, puddings should be an occasional treat and a fruit crumble made with fresh apple or rhubarb or frozen berries with an oat-based crumble is far better than a chocolate pudding with chocolate sauce. Cut down on fast-releasing, high-GL fruits like bananas or combine them with slow-releasing, low-GL carbohydrates such as oats. You can sweeten cereal with fruit and dilute fruit juices with water by at least half to halve their GL score. Avoid foods with added sugar. Read labels carefully – you're looking for '-oses' such as glucose, sucrose, maltose and dextrose.

## The exception to the rule

The one time when high-GL carbs are suitable for your child is if they have just done, or are about to do, some intense exercise, such as playing a game of football. A banana in the half-hour before the exercise works well, since any excess sugar will be used up quickly for energy. After exercise they'll need to boost their blood sugar levels fast, as not only will those blood sugar levels be low, but the glycogen storage units in the muscles and liver will also be depleted. Again, a high-GL snack such as a banana is ideal, because any excess glucose in the blood will go to replenish the empty glycogen stores, rather than building up into high blood sugar. Bananas are also a good source of potassium, which is lost in sweat.

Sports drinks are good for replenishing blood glucose and glycogen stores just before and after exercise, but you can easily make your own. Use 6g of maltodextrin powder, which is available in health food shops, mixed with 1 litre of water. The drink can be sipped in the half-hour before exercise, during breaks in games and training, and then when they've finished. A dash of salt can be added for older children, who will lose salt in their sweat. A home-made drink will be free from additives and colourings, and works out a lot cheaper, too.

## Stay away from sugar substitutes

While they won't raise blood sugar levels, sugar substitutes should not be part of your plan to cut down on sugar in your child's diet. Aspartame, the most widely used, is particularly bad and several studies have shown it to have adverse effects on children's health. One study into the effects of aspartame showed that it caused nightmares, memory loss, temper and nausea.[17] Apart from the dangers of additives, artificial sweeteners don't help children adjust to less sweet food either. For all of us, adults and children alike, staying away from sugar becomes easier and easier as our cravings for sugar subside, but sugar substitutes simply keep those cravings going. Furthermore, recent research on rats suggests that artificial sweeteners may even contribute to obesity.[18]

Having said that, there is one sugar substitute worth a mention: xylitol. It's derived from a natural source and is abundant in plums and cherries, which have a very low GL as a result. Compared with regular sugar or even fructose, xylitol has a fraction of the effect on blood sugar. For example, 9 teaspoons of xylitol has the same effect on the blood sugar as 4 teaspoons of fructose or 1 teaspoon of sugar. We still suggest you reduce your child's taste for sweet foods, but when some sweetness is really essential, for example, if you're whipping up dessert for a special occasion, then xylitol is the best alternative to sugar. Xylitol is readily available in all good health food shops and some supermarkets.

## The dynamic duo – protein and fibre

The more fibre and protein you include with any meal or snack, the slower the release of the carbohydrates. Fibre does the job by actually getting in the way of the carbohydrate, impeding its inter-action with digestive enzymes and effectively slowing its passage into the intestines, from where it is absorbed into the bloodstream. Protein, meanwhile, slows down the speed at which the stomach empties its contents of partially digested food into the intestines.

As we've seen, anything that slows the passage of carbohydrate into the bloodstream is good for your child's blood sugar balance, so combining protein-rich foods with high-fibre carbohydrates is an excellent rule of thumb in this context. Here's how you do it:

- Give seeds or nuts with a fruit snack

- Add seeds or nuts to carbohydrate-based breakfast cereals

- Serve salmon, chicken or lentils with brown basmati rice

- Add kidney beans to a pasta sauce served over wholemeal pasta

- Put cottage cheese on oatcakes or hummus on rye bread

- Make sandwiches with unsweetened peanut butter and wholemeal bread.

## Is it really juice?

Much of the 'fruit juice' on the market is not much better than sugary water. Once a fruit juice has been processed and put into a carton, it bears little resemblance to a fresh fruit juice in terms of colour, taste and nutrient content. Unfortunately, however, the sugar content remains intact. Children who regularly drink processed juice are taking in a lot of sugar and thereby messing up their blood sugar balance, feeding their sugar cravings, rotting their teeth and making themselves fat. Despite vigorous marketing to convince us to the contrary, the stuff in these cartons is not a good source of vitamins and minerals. Worst of all are the 'juice drinks', which almost invariably have added sugars and very little actual fruit juice.

However, this doesn't mean that juice is completely off the menu. You simply need to go for freshly squeezed or, failing that, chill-cabinet juices. These are obviously fresher, but be vigilant about checking the use-by date. If this is longer than just a few days into the future, we recommend you don't touch it. If it is expected to 'go off' in a few days, then it was probably reasonably nutritious when it went into the carton, but its nutrient content is declining by the hour. So inevitably, fruit that's juiced right in front of you is the best bet.

Along with freshness, you need to look at the GL score of various juices. Apple juice and pear juice are best, followed by orange. As we mentioned above, it's also important to dilute the juice your child drinks with water, as adding half a glass of water halves the GL score. Fresh vegetable juices can be drunk without dilution, with the possible exception of carrot juice.

The best drink for your child is water, so make this the staple and keep juice as an occasional treat. Children who are used to drinking nothing but juice or soft drinks will find water 'boring' to begin with, so ease them into it slowly. Before you know it, though, they'll find 'full-strength' juice unpalatable.

## Don't go without breakfast

Getting the kids up on a school morning with enough time for them to eat a decent breakfast can be challenging at the best of times, but eating a decent breakfast really is essential if your child is going to concentrate at school. If their blood sugar stays rock-bottom all morning, they'll be lethargic, irritable, lacking in focus and craving a sticky bun.

In one study, 29 schoolchildren were given different breakfast cereals, a glucose drink or no breakfast on different days. Their attention and memory were tested before breakfast, and again 30, 90, 150 and 210 minutes later. Children who had had the glucose drink or no breakfast showed poorer attention and memory compared to the children eating cereal.[19]

We find that children who eat a nutritious diet generally get a much better night's sleep, too (see chapter 17 for more on this). The knock-on effect is that it's easier for them to get out of bed in the morning, which in turn gives them the time and inclination to eat a decent breakfast, and they don't fall asleep in the classroom!

If your child doesn't have much of an appetite in the morning and frequently skips breakfast, help them by easing them into the habit gradually. Begin by giving them one strawberry. The next day make it two strawberries and a brazil nut or a teaspoon of sunflower seeds. The next day, half an apple and three almonds, and so on until after a couple of weeks they'll be able to eat a bowl of oats (as porridge, raw or lightly toasted) with fruit and nuts. Remember that you, too, need to eat breakfast! If you typically go to work on a cup of coffee, don't be surprised if your children attempt to imitate you.

## Caffeine affects blood sugar, too

Sugar isn't the only factor involved in blood sugar problems. Other stimulants – and caffeine is a powerful one – can also have a highly disruptive effect on your child's blood sugar balance. Caffeine is also an appetite suppressant and can be part of behaviours such as picky eating or refusing to contemplate breakfast. Supermarket shelves groan with products containing caffeine, though, so let's look at the most serious culprits.

### Cola and energy drinks

These contain anything from 46 to 80mg of caffeine per can, which is as much as you'd find in a regular cup of filter coffee. These drinks are often high in sugar and colourings, too, and their net stimulant effect can be considerable. Check the label on all canned drinks and keep your children away from any that contain caffeine and chemical additives or colourings. Also watch out for 'natural' stimulants such as guarana, because these have the same effect as caffeine.

### Chocolate bars and drinks

Chocolate bars are usually full of sugar, which is bad enough for the levels of glucose in your child's blood, but cocoa, the active ingredient in chocolate and in chocolate drinks, also provides significant quantities of the stimulant theobromine, which has a similar effect to caffeine, although it isn't as strong. Chocolate also contains small amounts of caffeine.

As chocolate is high in sugar and stimulants, reserve it as a special treat for your child. That means a small amount once a week rather than every day. Also bear in mind the relative sizes of the chocolate bar and your child. For example, don't give a toddler more than a square or two of chocolate at one sitting.

## Tea

In the UK, some people start their children off on the great British addiction very young indeed. Yet a strong cup of tea contains as much caffeine as a weak cup of coffee and is certainly addictive. Tea also contains tannin, which interferes with the absorption of vital minerals such as iron and zinc. Even 'decaffeinated' tea is not actually caffeine-free. The amount of caffeine in it is reduced, but the tannin levels remain the same.

If you want to give your child a hot drink, the best alternatives to tea are red bush (*rooibos*) tea with or without milk and herbal or fruit teas. Since these are naturally caffeine-free, they have no downsides. Older children can drink green tea, which has very low levels of caffeine and the natural catechins it contains are fantastic antioxidants, with numerous reported health benefits.

## Coffee

Coffee just becomes more and more popular and, again, many children are taking up the habit at a young age. Coffee contains three stimulants – caffeine, theobromine and theophylline. Although caffeine is the strongest of the three, theobromine, as we've said, has a similar effect to caffeine, although it's present in much smaller amounts in coffee than in cocoa, and theophylline is known to disturb normal sleep patterns.

So there's a host of stimulants in coffee waiting to mess up your child's blood sugar balance, but that's not all. It is also addictive and, despite general public perception, it actually worsens mental performance. Research published in the *American Journal of Psychiatry* studied 1,500 psychology students and found that moderate and high consumers of coffee were found to have higher levels of anxiety and depression than abstainers, and that the high consumers had the greatest incidence of stress-related medical problems, as well as lower academic performance.[20] A number of studies have shown that the ability to remember lists of words is made worse by caffeine, so children who drink coffee before school, especially as a pre-exam boost, are more likely to struggle in class.

The reason people get hooked on caffeine, particularly in the morning, is that it seems to make you feel better, more energised and alert. However, Dr Peter Rogers, a psychologist at Bristol University, wondered whether caffeine actually increases your energy and mental performance or just relieves the symptoms of withdrawal. When he researched this he found that, after that sacred cup of coffee, coffee drinkers don't feel any better than people who never drink coffee – they just feel better than they did when they woke up.[21] So the important message here is don't let your children start drinking coffee. It isn't good for them and, like any addiction, giving up becomes more difficult the longer you have the habit.

Like decaffeinated tea, decaffeinated coffee isn't stimulant-free, because only some of the caffeine is removed and the other stimulants remain. The most popular alternatives are Teeccino, Caro, Barley Cup, dandelion coffee or herbal teas. If your child already has the taste for coffee, offer a choice of these substitutes. They may experience 'withdrawal' symptoms when they give up coffee, such as headaches, but these will disappear within a few days.

## Summary

To ensure your child's blood sugar levels remain balanced and even:

- Choose wholefoods – wholegrains, lentils, beans, nuts, seeds, fresh fruit and vegetables. With fruit and veg, go for dark green, leafy and root vegetables, such as watercress, carrots, sweet potatoes, broccoli, Brussels sprouts, spinach, green beans or peppers, raw or lightly cooked. Choose fresh fruit such as apples, pears, berries, melon or citrus fruit and, infrequently, bananas. Provide five or more servings of fruit and vegetables each day.

- Avoid overly processed foods.

- Choose wholegrains such as rice, buckwheat, millet, rye, oats, wholewheat, corn or quinoa in cereal, breads and pasta. Avoid refined 'white' foods.

- Avoid sugar and foods containing sugar. This means anything with '-ose' at the end, including glucose, sucrose, dextrose and maltose. Don't be tempted to go for sugar substitutes as most are detrimental to health and they all keep sugar cravings alive.

- Combine protein foods with carbohydrate foods by giving cereals and fruit with nuts or seeds, and ensuring your child eats carbohydrate-rich foods, such as potatoes, bread, pasta, or rice, with protein-rich foods, such as fish, chicken, lentils, beans or eggs. As fibre is important for slowing sugar absorption, make sure your child is getting ample fibre in fruit and veg.

continues →

- Choose real fresh fruit juices from the chill cabinet and dilute them half and half with water. Steer clear of the highly processed kind of fruit juice with a long shelf-life. Make water the staple drink.

- Encourage your child to eat breakfast.

- Help your child avoid caffeinated food and drinks, such as chocolate, tea, coffee and 'energy' drinks.

# Chapter 3

•

# Fats – the good, the bad and the ugly

Unfortunately, fat has such a bad name it's almost a four-letter word. However, fats are an important component of your child's diet – at least the right fats are. Put simply, there are three types of fats: the good fats – polyunsaturated oils from seeds, nuts and oily fish (otherwise known as omega-3 and omega-6 fats); the bad fats – saturated fats from meat, eggs and dairy, although these are only bad if your child eats too much of them; and the ugly – the trans fats found in processed foods and fried foods. There's also olive oil, which, technically speaking, is in a category of its own, because it's a good fat, but isn't quite in the league of the omega-3 and omega-6 fats.

## The good fats

Essential fats – the omega-3 and omega-6 essential fats – help children stay physically healthy, reducing the risk of allergies, asthma, eczema and infections, due to their anti-inflammatory and immune-supportive properties. Every single cell of the human body is held together by a thin membrane which is composed of fats, primarily the essential fats. The composition of fats in this membrane is determined by the composition of the fats that your child eats. Due to their physical shape, essential fats contribute to a better quality cell membrane, which allows nutrients and oxygen to get into the cell more easily, and helps carbon dioxide and other waste products leave the cell efficiently.

More than this, they promote mental health, too. A deficiency can result in fatigue, memory, behavioural and developmental problems, depression, dyslexia, attention deficit disorder and autism.

## CASE HISTORY *Adrian, age 3*

Adrian was brought to the Brain Bio Centre by his parents, because they were concerned about his loss of speech development. They had already put him on a dairy- and gluten-free diet and were pleased to see that his eczema had disappeared and his asthma had improved dramatically. We ran some tests which showed he was very low in magnesium, selenium and zinc, and also in essential fats. We recommended a fish oil, multivitamin and mineral supplement. Within days of starting the fish oil, Adrian began to chatter again.

The bottom line is that essential fats really *are* essential for keeping your child healthy and these fats are also needed in optimal amounts to maximise your child's intelligence. We use the word 'intelligence' very broadly here. Your child's ability to perform in the world depends on a balance of mental, emotional and physical intelligence. Most people are aware of mental intelligence, because the IQ tests that determine a person's ability to make intellectual connections and deal with complex concepts are well known, but emotional intelligence is no less important. Your child's EQ is a measure of his or her ability to respond emotionally to situations in an appropriate and sensitive way. If they lose their temper easily, and switch rapidly between depression and hyperactivity, lacking emotional balance and perspective, there's room for improvement – however 'bright' they may be. Then there's physical intelligence. PQ is all about brain–body coordination. For example, children with a low PQ may seem clumsy and uncoordinated or have trouble with skills such as handwriting, reading and taking notes in class.

## Never too late to start

Every type of intelligence – IQ, EQ and PQ – is affected by your child's intake of omega-3s and omega-6s. Children deficient in essential fats have more learning difficulties, while children who are breast-fed have higher IQs at age eight than bottle-fed babies, which is thought to be due to the higher levels of essential fats in breast milk.[1–2]

Studies by Dr Peter Willatts at the University of Dundee in Scotland showed that babies fed a formula enriched with a specific essential fat (DHA) had better problem-solving skills at ten months of age.[3] Also, giving omega-3 essential fats to pregnant and breast-feeding women has been shown to improve their children's intellectual function right up until the children are four.[4] Research is currently underway that is likely to show that these benefits persist into adulthood.

Essential fats remain important throughout life, so your child will continue to need them as they grow, but the good news is that it's never too late to boost your child's levels of essential fats. For example, research by Dr Alex Richardson at Oxford University has proven the value of essential fats in a trial involving 41 children aged eight to 12 years who had symptoms of attention deficit hyperactivity disorder (ADHD) and specific learning difficulties. Those children receiving extra essential fats in supplements were both behaving and learning better within 12 weeks.[5] Another trial by Dr Richardson showed significant improvement in reading ability in children on essential fats supplements, compared with children taking a placebo, over six months.[6] All this confirms American surveys carried out at Purdue University that showed children with ADHD tend to get lower levels of essential fats than children without ADHD.[7] Giving essential fats supplements was found to reduce ADHD symptoms such as anxiety, attention difficulties and general behaviour problems.[8-9]

To date, much of the research on essential fats has focused on their benefits to behavioural and developmental health, but they help keep your child in good physical health, too. Essential fats are processed by the body into eicosanoids. These are special molecules that act as messengers in the central nervous system and are involved in many bodily processes, mainly relating to inflammation or immunity, so the quantity of essential fats in the diet affects inflammatory processes in the body.[10] There are several families of eicosanoids, some of which help cause inflammation – anti-inflammatory drugs such as aspirin slow the production of pro-inflammatory eicosanoids – and some of which work to stop inflammation – those derived from omega-3 fats are generally anti-inflammatory.

Most diseases, including allergies, are associated with inflammation. In one study, Korean researchers investigated whether the essential fats played a role in allergies in children. The team took a measure of essential fats in the red blood cells of 308 children aged between four and six years old and compared this to the prevalence of allergic symptoms, such as dermatitis, hay fever and asthma. The children with the most symptoms were those with the lowest levels of the essential fats, particularly the omega-3 fats EPA and DHA that are found in oily fish.[11]

The essential fats also keep your child 'well-oiled', contributing to soft, smooth skin and silky, glossy hair. So, while it seems such a simple thing, upping your child's essential fat intake can have profound benefits for their health.

**FAT CHECK**

Check your child's intake of essential fats by answering the questions below:

Does your child...

☐ eat oily fish, such as salmon, trout, sardines, herring, mackerel or fresh tuna, less than once a week?

☐ eat seeds or their cold-pressed oils fewer than three times a week?

☐ eat meat or dairy products most days?

☐ eat processed or fried foods (such as ready meals, chips or crisps) three or more times a week?

☐ have dry or rough skin or a tendency to eczema?

☐ have dry or dull hair or dandruff?

☐ suffer from dry, watery or itchy eyes?

☐ suffer from excessive thirst or frequent urination?

☐ have frequent mood swings?

☐ have a poor memory, attention span or difficulty concentrating?

☐ have poor physical coordination?

*If you answer 'yes' to five or more of these questions, the chances are your child isn't getting enough essential fats.*

Ultimately, however, the most precise way to know your child's essential fat status is to have a blood test. This is what we do at the Brain Bio Centre and other nutritional therapists offer them, too. The test gives you a complete breakdown of all the essential fats in your child's body and shows which ones are lacking.

## Go to school on an egg

Similar to saturated fats, a moderate amount of cholesterol in the diet is perfectly acceptable and even necessary. Cholesterol is used to make the body's chemical messengers – hormones – and it's also an important component of cell membranes. How good or bad it is depends on how it's cooked. Overcooked, fried or burnt cholesterol is bad for your child's health, so don't char meat or fry bacon and eggs until they're crispy.

In fact, as long as you don't fry it, a free-range, organic, omega-3-rich egg is a veritable superfood and if you lightly boil, hardboil, poach or gently scramble them you can safely give your child six to ten eggs a week. People these days, however, are often egg-phobic, believing that eggs are unhealthy, due to their high fat and cholesterol content. This just isn't true, particularly as some fat and cholesterol are essential for health, especially for children. The kind of fat you find in an egg depends on what you feed the chicken. If you feed them a diet rich in omega-3s, for example flaxseeds or fishmeal, you get an egg high in omega-3s. An egg is as healthy as the chicken that laid it. As for cholesterol, it's simply a myth that what you find in eggs is bad for your child or you – it will neither raise blood cholesterol nor cause heart disease.

Eggs are also a great source of something called phospholipids, which are the special 'intelligent' fats in our brains. They are insulation experts, helping make up the myelin sheath, which covers all our nerves, promoting a smooth run for signals in the brain. Phospholipids, which are not only found in eggs, but also in fish, especially sardines, organic meats and, to a lesser extent, soya and nuts – make the brain 'sing', enhancing your child's mood, mind and mental performance.

## PHOSPHOLIPID CHECK

Check your child's intake of phospholipids by answering the questions below:

Does your child...

☐ eat fish less than once a week?

☐ eat fewer than three eggs per week?

☐ eat soya, tofu or nuts less than three times per week?

☐ take less than 5g of lecithin each day?

☐ have a poor memory?

☐ find it hard to do calculations in their head?

☐ sometimes have difficulty concentrating?

☐ have a tendency toward depression?

☐ appear to be a 'slow learner'?

*If you answer 'yes' to five or more of these questions, the chances are your child isn't getting enough phospholipids.*

To increase the phospholipid-rich foods in your child's diet, give them perhaps an egg a day, sardines twice a week or organic liver once a week. Phospholipids are often part of brain food formulas and a daily supplement can really help some children with poor memories (see chapter 25 for more on this). Lecithin is another good supplement source of phospholipids and is widely available in health food shops, where it's sold either as lecithin granules or capsules. The easiest and cheapest way to take this is to add a tablespoon of lecithin or a heaped teaspoon of high-PC (phosphatidyl choline) lecithin to your child's cereal in the morning.

# And now the bad

In all honesty we're reluctant to call saturated fats the bad fats. It's true that if you eat too much fat, it can make you fat, but, as we saw in the previous chapter, for most children who are overweight the biggest culprit is likely to be sugar, and indeed the trans fats which we'll come to shortly.

Saturated fats are typically solid at room temperature and are mostly found in food from animal sources, such as meat, dairy produce and eggs. Coconut oil and avocados also contain saturated fat. Children, in particular, need some of this fat in their daily diet, partly for use as energy and partly to be incorporated into their bodies as they grow. Saturated fat is not technically essential in the diet, because the body can manufacture what it needs from the essential fats, but it doesn't make sense for a child to avoid it altogether, even if they're overweight, because fatty foods provide fat-soluble vitamins such as vitamins A, D and E (see chapter 5 for more on this).

A good use of saturated fats is for frying. Saturated fats are not damaged by heat and converted into trans fats in the way that the polyunsaturated fats, such as the omega fats, are. So we suggest using butter or virgin coconut oil if you're frying food at home. Always fry at the lowest possible temperature to reduce the amount of oxidants you create (see chapter 6 for more on this).

## Olive oil – the special case

Monounsaturated fats, which include olive oil, are liquid at room temperature, but will start solidifying if refrigerated (the omega fats and other polyunsaturates remain liquid even at much lower temperatures). Olive oil features heavily in the Mediterranean diet and there is plenty of evidence that good-quality olive oil contributes to health, so use it liberally for salad dressings. Virgin olive oil is best eaten raw as cooking with it will produce some trans fats. If you must fry with olive oil, use the medium or mild varieties as these are less prone to damage and always fry at the lowest possible temperatures to avoid damaging the fats.

# Finally, the 'ugly'

The worst fats your child can eat are the trans fats. These fats are damaged fats found in deep-fried food and foods containing hydrogenated vegetable oils. These fats are so bad that they have been banned in Scandinavian countries (bar trace amounts that occur naturally) for some years now. Since January 2006, they must be declared on labels in the US and Canada. Sadly, in the UK the Food Standards Agency (FSA) has been rather slow to recognise the dangers of trans fats to the public's health. The FSA continues to focus on saturated fats as the bad guy, despite strong evidence that many, if not all, the negative health effects associated with saturated fats are much more strongly associated with trans fats. For example, trans fats are worse for heart disease and they're worse for making people fat. Trans fats also block the conversion of essential fats into vital brain fats, such as GLA and DHA.

So a combined deficiency in omega-3 fats and an excess of trans fats – the hallmark of the chicken-nugget-and-fries generation – is a bad scenario. A serving of chips or fried fish can each deliver 8g of trans fats, a doughnut 12g and a bag of crisps more than 4g.

So, how do you root out trans fats when they're not declared on food labels. Firstly, trans fats rarely occur in natural foods and when they do they are relatively harmless and the amounts are miniscule. They are created when food is fried, especially deep-fried, and often in the processing of food, so limiting fried and processed food will cut most of them out of your child's diet. Trans fats are widely used to extend shelf life, which is why food manufacturers love them. If a food label lists any type of fat as an ingredient and has a long shelf-life, for example a cake or muffin that has an expiry date six months in the future, it probably contains trans fats. The ideal amount of trans fats in your child's diet is zero.

# Fat figures

So how much of the various fats will your child need to stay mentally and physically healthy? To answer that we first need to look at the optimal amount of overall fat in their diet. It's best to consume no more than 20 per cent of all calories as fat. The current average in Britain is around 40 per cent. In countries with a low incidence of heart disease and other fat-related diseases, such Japan, Thailand and the Philippines, people consume only about 15 per cent of their total calorie intake as fat.

Most authorities now agree that, of our total fat intake, no more than a third should be saturated fat and at least a third should be polyunsaturated oils providing the two essential fats, omega-3 and omega-6. These two essential fat families also need to be in balance, in a rough ratio of 1:1, which is what our ancestors were getting before the Industrial Revolution. Then, people ate local foods with an abundance of seeds, whereas the widespread exodus to the cities resulted in the rise of easily stored refined foods and hard fats. Nowadays the balance is more like 1:20 in favour of omega-6s.

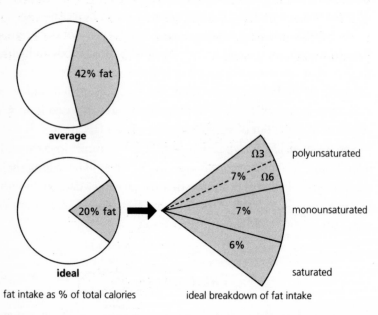

*What we eat vs what we need*

Consequently, it may not just be the gross deficiency in omega-3 fats that has led to so many of the health problems we see in children today, but also the gross imbalance between the two omegas. In addition, a high intake of saturated fats and trans fats stops the body from making good use of the little essential fat the average person does eat in a day.

## The omega-3s

By now you'll have gathered how important the omega fat families are to your child's health. Let's delve deeper, first taking a closer look at the essential fats so many children lack – the omega-3s.

Why is the modern-day diet likely to be more deficient in omega-3 fats than in omega-6s? It's all because the 'grandmother' of the omega-3 family, alpha-linolenic acid, and her metabolically active 'grandchildren' eicosapentaenoic acid (EPA) and docosahexaenoic acid (DHA), are more unsaturated and so more prone to damage by cooking, heating and food processing. For example, if you fry a piece of fish or roast seeds, you will actually damage some of the omega-3s they contain. In any event, the average person today eats a mere sixth of the omega-3 fats found in the

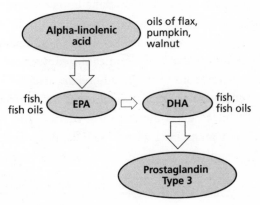

*Omega-3 fat family*

average European diet of 1850. This decline is partly due to food choices, but mainly due to food processing.

Alpha-linolenic acid is abundant in cold-climate seeds, such as flaxseeds, and also plankton, the vegetation of the sea. Our bodies can convert some of this alpha-linolenic acid into EPA and DHA, but a more effective way to increase supplies of these more 'active' omega-3s is to eat oily fish. This is because the fish has already done the conversion for us in its own body. The primary source of EPA and DHA is coldwater fish, especially fish that eat fish, such as herring, mackerel, salmon and fresh tuna. Sardines are also an excellent source.

However, there are a few caveats here. Since canned tuna has much less omega-3, stick with fresh tuna, but because larger fish such as tuna tend to contain more mercury, which they have absorbed when swimming in polluted water, don't feed tuna steaks to your child more than twice a month and less if you're concerned about mercury toxicity (see chapter 6 for more on this). As for salmon, the amount of EPA and DHA in the farmed fish really depends on the quality of its diet and, as with most intensive farming practices this can be variable. Organic farmed or wild salmon is much better in this respect.

As a rule of thumb, children normally need around 300 to 400mg of both DHA and EPA a day (see chapter 25 for more on this). The conversion in the body of alpha-linolenic acid in, say, flax (linseeds) and pumpkin seeds, to EPA and DHA can be very inefficient. For this reason, vegetarians rarely have sufficient levels of EPA and DHA unless they eat significant quantities of flaxseeds, which are the richest source of alpha-linolenic acid.

So during critical periods of development such as childhood, it may be preferable to get a direct source of EPA and DHA from fish, backed up by an indirect supply from flaxseeds or flaxseed oil. This would certainly be recommended for a pregnant or breast-feeding woman to allow her to pass on sufficient EPA and DHA to her child. The World Health Organization now recommends that formula feeds include these oils.[12] DHA is especially important during the foetal stage and infancy, because it is literally used to build the brain and makes up a full quarter of the brain's dry weight.

In many cases, children with learning and behavioural problems are even less efficient than the average child at converting alpha-linolenic acid into EPA and DHA. Partly for this reason, a child with ADHD or dyslexia may need double or triple their intake to help their condition.

From the point of view of omega-3 fats, the best diet is 'fishitar-ian', where your child eats fish three times a week; or, failing that, a seed-rich vegan diet. Eggs can also provide significant quantities of omega-3 if the hens were fed a high-omega-3 diet – check the egg box labels. Remember, though, not only is it important to eat a rich direct source of omega-3 fats such as fish, or a rich indirect source such as flaxseeds, it's also vital for your child to go easy on the saturated fat and avoid processed fat.

## The omega-6s

Your child will also need omega-6 fats and the 'grandmother' of the omega-6 fat family is linoleic acid, which is found in hot-climate seeds such as sunflower and sesame seeds. Linoleic acid is converted by the body into gamma-linolenic acid (GLA), which may be familiar to you as a substance in evening primrose oil and borage or starflower oil, which are the richest known sources. A derivative of GLA, known as DGLA, is found in high quantities in the brain.

Giving children supplementary GLA, usually through evening primrose oil, has proven effective in alleviating a wide variety of health problems. For example, a study on children with dyspraxia showed that essential fats supplements, including omega-6 oil, improved reading, writing and behaviour in just three months.[13]

However, one omega-6 fat has something of a Jekyll and Hyde nature and that's arachidonic acid (AA). While there's no question that it's an essential fat and a major component of the brain, in

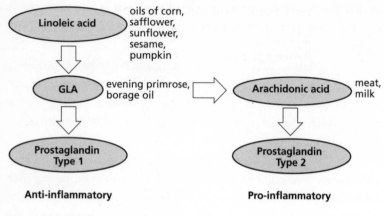

*Omega-6 fat family*

excess in the body arachidonic acid is bad news as it is can promote inflammation. It can be derived either directly from meat or animal produce, or indirectly from linoleic acid or GLA, but the latter may be a preferable source because GLA also produces anti-inflammatory substances that balance the inflammatory effects of arachidonic acid. For this and other reasons, to get enough of this essential fat family it's best to let your child eat omega-6-rich seeds and their oils, rather than overdosing on meat and dairy produce, especially if they have an inflammatory condition such as eczema, asthma or allergies.

## Where to get the omegas

As we've seen, the seeds with the highest levels of omega-3 fats are flax, although hemp and pumpkin seeds are rich sources, too. The only direct source of the essential omega-3 brain boosters EPA and DHA are oily fish. The best seeds for omega-6 fats are hemp, pumpkin, sunflower, safflower, sesame and maize kernels. Walnuts, soya beans and wheatgerm are also rich in omega-6s.

**BEST FOODS FOR ESSENTIAL FATS**

| Omega-3 | Omega-6 |
|---|---|
| Flaxseeds (linseed) | Corn |
| Hemp seed | Safflower |
| Pumpkin seeds | Sunflower |
|  | Sesame |
|  | Walnut |

| EPA and DHA | GLA |
|---|---|
| Salmon | Evening primrose oil |
| Mackerel | Borage oil |
| Herring | Blackcurrant seed |
| Sardines |  |
| Anchovies (whole, not salted fillets) |  |
| Tuna (steaks, not tinned) |  |
| Eggs (from flaxseed-fed hens) |  |

So what's the best way of incorporating these essential fats into your child's daily menu? There are three possibilities: seeds and fish; seed oils, which are more concentrated in essential fats, but don't provide other nutrients such as minerals, which are abundant in the whole seeds; or giving concentrated fish oils and seed oils, such as flax, evening primrose or starflower oil, as supplements.

## Seeds and fish

If you want to go with seeds, put one measure each of sesame, sunflower and pumpkin seeds, and three measures of flaxseeds, into a sealed jar. Keep it in the fridge, away from light, heat and oxygen. Simply adding one heaped tablespoon of these seeds, freshly ground in a coffee grinder, to your child's cereal each morning guarantees a good daily intake of essential fats. If your child is eating a hot cereal such as porridge for breakfast, add the seeds to the cooked porridge just before serving. We also recommend that your child eats 100g of oily fish (roughly equivalent in size to one tin of sardines or a mackerel fillet) two or three times a week.

## Seed oils

If you want to go with oils, the best place to start is an oil blend that offers a 1:1 ratio of omega-3 and omega-6 fats, is cold-pressed, preferably organic and kept refrigerated before you buy it. These are now widely available in health food stores (see Products and supplements directory). The oil can be added to salads and other cold or warm foods, but must not be heated. Some children will take it neat from the spoon. Hemp-seed oil is the next best thing. It provides 19 per cent alpha-linolenic acid (omega-3), 57 per cent linoleic acid and 2 per cent GLA (both omega-6s) (see chapter 25 for more on supplement levels for different ages).

## Supplements

As far as supplements are concerned, for omega-6 your best bet is starflower (borage) oil or evening primrose oil. Starflower oil provides more GLA and fish oils are best for omega-3. There are supplements that combine EPA, DHA and GLA. For smaller children who can't swallow pills or tablets, a number of supplements are available in liquid form and flavoured in various ways (see chapter 25 for more on supplement levels for different ages).

## Summary

To ensure your child gets the right kinds of fats:

- Provide plenty of seeds and nuts – the best seeds are flax, hemp, pumpkin, sunflower and sesame. You get more goodness out of them by grinding them first and sprinkling them on cereals, soups and salads.

continues →

- Choose coldwater carnivorous fish – a serving of sardines, mackerel, herring, kipper or wild or organic salmon two or three times a week provides a good source of omega-3 fats.

- Choose cold-pressed seed oils – either an oil blend or hemp oil for salad dressings and other cold uses.

- Avoid fried and processed food, and baked goods with a long shelf life.

- Choose fish oil to supplement omega-3 fats and starflower or evening primrose oil for omega-6 fats.

- Add a tablespoon of lecithin granules or a heaped teaspoon of high-PC lecithin to your child's cereal every day.

- Or give your child an egg for breakfast – preferably a free-range, organic egg that's high in omega-3s and lightly boiled or scrambled, but definitely not fried.

- Or give your child a brain food formula supplement providing phosphatidyl choline and phosphatidyl serine, especially if your child is having learning problems (see chapter 9 for more on this).

# Chapter 4

·

# Protein power

Protein provides your child with amino acids – the building blocks of life. The word protein itself is derived from *protos*, a Greek word meaning 'first', since protein is the basic material of all living cells. The human body, for example, contains approximately 25 per cent protein.

Just as a sentence is made up of words and words of letters, protein is made up of peptides and peptides are made up of amino acids. When your child eats protein-rich foods such as meat, eggs, fish, dairy, lentils, beans or quinoa (an Andean grain, pronounced 'keen-wa'), their digestive system breaks down the protein first into peptides and then into amino acids. By linking amino acids together in different sequences, their body then builds up new muscle or organ tissue, enzymes or neurotransmitters – the chemical messengers of the brain. A good supply of protein, and hence of amino acids, will keep your child well supplied with the building blocks that make growth and development possible, plus, as we've already seen, protein plays a key role in supporting good blood sugar balance, too.

## AMINO ACID CHECK

Check your child's amino acid levels by answering the questions below:

Does your child...

- [ ] eat less than one portion of protein-rich foods, such as meat, dairy, fish, eggs or pulses, each day?

- [ ] eat fewer than two servings of vegetable sources of protein, such as beans, lentils, quinoa, seeds, nuts, wholegrains and so on, each day?

- [ ] if they're vegetarian, do they rarely combine different protein foods such as those mentioned above?

- [ ] engage in a lot of physical activity?

- [ ] suffer from anxiety, depression or irritability?

- [ ] seem to be frequently tired or lack motivation?

- [ ] sometimes lose concentration or have poor memory?

- [ ] have slow-growing hair and nails?

- [ ] seem to be constantly hungry?

- [ ] frequently get indigestion?

*If you answer 'yes' to five or more of these questions, the chances are your child isn't getting enough amino acids.*

Upping your child's intake of protein can make all the difference. Read on to discover how to boost your child's protein intake and boost their mental and physical energy.

# Protein balance

The quality of a protein is determined by its balance of amino acids. Although there are 23 amino acids which the body can use to build anything from a neurotransmitter to a muscle cell, only eight are known as essential, because they must be obtained through diet. If there is not enough of the other 15 in the diet, they can be made in the body from the essential eight. However, in children, some amino acids are known as semi-essential, because children may not be able to manufacture adequate quantities of them.

A child needs to eat between one or two 20g servings of protein a day, depending on their age:

**PROTEIN REQUIREMENT BY AGE**

|  | 2–3 years | 4–8 years | 9–13 years | 14–18 years (girls) | 14–18 years (boys) |
| --- | --- | --- | --- | --- | --- |
| Protein | 13g | 19g | 34g | 46g | 52g |

The better the balance of amino acids in a protein – expressed as its 'net protein usability' (NPU) – the more you can make use of that protein. The chart opposite shows the top 24 individual foods and food combinations in terms of NPUs or protein quality. Combining lentils or beans with rice, for example, is a great way of increasing the overall quality of the protein, because lentils and beans are rich in the amino acids rice is low in. The chart also shows how much of a food, or a food combination, you need to eat to get a 20g serving of protein.

A typical day's protein for a six-year-old might therefore include two of any of the following: an egg (10g), a 50g serving of salmon, a handful (60g) of seeds and nuts, or a serving of beans (100g).

For a vegetarian child, a typical day's worth might be any two of the following: a small tub of yoghurt, a handful of seeds or nuts, a 140g serving of tofu, a small cup of quinoa or a small serving of

beans with rice. The trick for vegetarians is to eat 'seed' foods –
foods that would grow if you planted them – like nuts, beans,
lentils, peas, maize or the germ of grains such as wheat or oat.
'Flower' foods such as broccoli or cauliflower are also relatively
rich in protein.

## PACKED WITH PROTEIN: THE TOP 24

| Food | Percentage of calories as protein | How much provides 20g of protein | Protein quality (NPU) |
|---|---|---|---|
| **Grains and pulses** | | | |
| Quinoa | 16 | 100g/1 cup dry weight | Excellent |
| Tofu | 40 | 275g/1 packet | Reasonable |
| Maize | 4 | 500g/3 cups cooked weight | Reasonable |
| Brown rice | 5 | 400g/3 cups cooked weight | Excellent |
| Chickpeas | 22 | 115g/$^2$/3 cup cooked weight | Reasonable |
| Lentils | 28 | 85g/1 cup cooked weight | Reasonable |
| **Fish and meat** | | | |
| Tuna, tinned | 61 | 85g/1 small tin | Excellent |
| Cod | 60 | 35g/1 very small piece | Excellent |
| Salmon | 50 | 100g/1 small piece | Excellent |
| Sardines | 49 | 100g/1 baked | Excellent |
| Chicken | 63 | 75g/1 small roasted breast | Excellent |
| **Nuts and seeds** | | | |
| Sunflower seeds | 15 | 185g/1 cup | Reasonable |
| Pumpkin seeds | 21 | 75g/$^1$/2 cup | Reasonable |
| Cashew nuts | 12 | 115g/1 cup | Reasonable |
| Almonds | 13 | 115g/1 cup | Reasonable |
| **Eggs and dairy** | | | |
| Eggs | 34 | 115g/2 medium | Excellent |
| Yoghurt, natural | 22 | 450g/3 small pots | Excellent |
| Cottage cheese | 49 | 125g/1 small pot | Excellent |

continues →

| Food | Percentage of calories as protein | How much provides 20g of protein | Protein quality (NPU) |
|---|---|---|---|
| **Vegetables** | | | |
| Peas, frozen | 26 | 250g/2 cups | Reasonable |
| Other beans | 20 | 200g/2 cups | Reasonable |
| Broccoli | 50 | 40g/½ cup | Reasonable |
| Spinach | 49 | 40g/⅔ cup | Reasonable |
| **Combinations** | | | |
| Lentils and rice | 18 | 125g/small cup dry weight | Excellent |
| Beans and rice | 15 | 125g/small cup dry weight | Excellent |

Cup measures are imperial.

Be aware, though, that more doesn't always mean better and your child can have too much protein. Although it does depend on your child's current growth pattern, exercise level and hence their need for protein, a daily protein intake of more than 85g a day can have negative health consequences. For instance, the breakdown products of protein, such as ammonia, are toxic to the body and eliminating them puts the kidneys under stress. Also, too many amino acids mean too much acid in the blood, which the body neutralises by releasing calcium from bone. Indeed it is now well established that diets very high in protein contribute to kidney disease and osteoporosis, so, as with all else in nutrition, balance is important.

Extreme protein deficiency, characterised by a pot belly with skinny arms and legs, is rarely seen in the developed world. However, deficiency in amino acids isn't at all uncommon and can give rise to depression, apathy and lack of motivation, an inability to relax, and poor memory and concentration. Supplementing specific amino acids has been proven to correct all these problems. For example, a form of the amino acid tryptophan has proven more effective in trials than the best antidepressant drugs,[1] the amino acid tyrosine improves mental and physical performance under stress better than coffee[2] and GABA is highly effective against anxiety.[3]

# Key players in the orchestra of mind

To understand why amino acids are so important for your child's brain, though, we first need to explore what the neurotransmitters or chemical messengers they build actually do. There are hundreds of different kinds of neurotransmitters in the brain and body, but here are the main players.

## The most important neurotransmitters

- **Adrenalin, noradrenalin and dopamine** make us feel good, stimulating and motivating us and helping us deal with stress.

- **GABA** counteracts these stimulating neurotransmitters by relaxing us and calming us down after stress.

- **Serotonin** keeps us happy, improving our mood and banishing the blues.

- **Acetylcholine** keeps our brain sharp, improving memory and mental alertness.

- **Tryptamines** keep us connected so, for example, melatonin keeps us in sync with day and night and the seasons.

Many other substances in the brain, such as endorphins, which give us a sense of euphoria after exercise, act much like neuro-transmitters, but those listed above are the big five and your child's mood, memory and mental alertness are all affected by their activity. If your child's serotonin is up, for example, they are likely to be happy; if dopamine and adrenalin are down, they are likely to feel unmotivated and tired. Having the right balance of these key neurotransmitters is a must if you want your child to be in tip-top mental health.

Amino acids do the job in a very similar way to that of pre-scribed drugs that directly affect neurotransmitters. For instance, amphetamines such as Ritalin work by causing an excessive release of adrenalin, whereas antidepressants like Seroxat (an SSRI) effectively raise levels of serotonin by preventing its breakdown in the body. These drugs have many undesirable side-effects, though, essentially working against our body's natural design, not with it, and SSRI antidepressants have rather fallen out of favour, particularly for use in children, as more and more studies show the benefits do not outweigh the risks.

Nutrients such as amino acids work just as well, if not better, but don't have the side-effects. After all, it's part of the brain and body's natural design to use them. So the best way to tune up your child's brain is to ensure they have an adequate intake of amino acids in their diet. First and foremost, this means eating enough protein every day and, to support good blood sugar balance, which is also vital for good emotional balance, some protein should be included with every meal and snack.

## Supplementing amino acids

If your child is eating a reasonable amount of protein, they should be getting all the amino acids that they need, but if they are having particular problems with mood or memory, you could consider supplements (see part 3 for more on this). Tests to measure levels of amino acids are available through nutritional therapists (see Resources), who, based on the results, may then recommend that your child takes particular amino acids in supplement form.

### Summary

To ensure your child is getting enough protein power:

- Give them between one and two servings of the protein-rich foods shown in the table on page 51 every day, depending on their age.

continues →

- Include some protein with every meal, such as chickpeas or chicken in their pasta sauce or nuts and seeds with their cereal. This is essential for blood sugar balance.

- Choose good vegetable protein sources, including beans, lentils, quinoa, tofu and 'seed' vegetables such as broccoli.

- If your child eats animal protein, choose free-range eggs, fish or lean meat, and go for organic whenever possible.

## Chapter 5

·

# Vital vitamins and magic minerals

We've talked about the big players – carbohydrates, fats and proteins – known as macronutrients. They make up the bulk of your child's diet and the bulk of your child, and are all used to provide energy. Vitamins and minerals are known as micronutrients and if macronutrients are the brawn, vitamins and minerals are the brains. Without them, your child can't turn carbohydrates into energy, process essential fats or build amino acids from proteins into things like neurotransmitters. In short, they are key to the task of building and rebuilding your child's body and brain, and keeping everything running smoothly.

Vitamins are organic compounds, which means they are constructed of lots of elements, all joined together in various configurations. A single vitamin may have several names, for example alpha-tocopherol, gamma-tocopherol and tocotrienol are all forms of vitamin E. With the exception of vitamins D and K, vitamins must be eaten. Minerals, on the other hand, are a single element, known by a single name, which you will find on the periodic table of elements. For example, calcium, magnesium and zinc are minerals. We cannot make minerals; they must be obtained from our diet.

# Vital vitamins

Let's take a closer look at vitamins and their diverse range of functions in the body. They function as antioxidants, hormones, immune-mediators and coenzymes, which are helper molecules that help chemical reactions between other molecules to take place.

Vitamins are classified as either water-soluble or fat-soluble and this generally dictates whether you'll find them in watery or fatty foods. In humans there are 13 vitamins: four are fat-soluble (A, D, E and K) and nine water-soluble (eight B vitamins and vitamin C), with each vitamin having a multitude of functions.

The health value of eating certain foods was recognised long before vitamins were identified. The ancient Egyptians knew that feeding a patient liver would help cure night blindness, an illness now known to be caused by a vitamin A deficiency. Liver, of course, is rich in vitamin A. In the 1700s, the Scottish surgeon James Lind discovered that citrus foods helped prevent scurvy, a particularly deadly disease in which collagen is not properly formed, causing poor wound healing, bleeding of the gums, severe pain and death. In this way a severe vitamin C deficiency disease, which took the lives of many sailors of the time, was avoided by regular consumption of vitamin C-rich lemons and limes.

Overt vitamin deficiency diseases, such as scurvy, are virtually unheard of in the developed world today, but sub-clinical deficiency of many vitamins is common. Vitamins are delicate molecules that can be destroyed to varying degrees by light, heat and oxygen, so the longer a food sits around or the more that is 'done' to it, such as cooking and processing, the lower the vitamin content will be. Intensive farming methods, such as harvesting fruit before it's ripe, means than many hitherto vitamin-rich foods may lack these wonderful nutrients. Much of the food that's eaten in the modern world has been processed, packaged or otherwise adulterated, or stored for too long, so the vitamin content may be further depleted.

## Magic minerals

More than a hundred years ago a Russian chemist called Mendelyeff noticed that all the basic constituents of matter, the elements, could be arranged in a pattern according to their chemical properties. From this he produced what is known as the periodic table. There were many gaps where elements should be and, sure enough, over the years these missing elements have been discovered. All matter, including your and your child's body, is made out of these elements.

Some of these are gases, like oxygen and hydrogen; some are liquids; and some, such as iron, zinc and chromium, are solids. Ninety-six per cent of the body is made up of carbon, hydrogen, oxygen and nitrogen, which form carbohydrate, protein and fat, as well as vitamins. The remaining 4 per cent is made from minerals.

Minerals are extracted from the soil in the first place by plants. Like vitamins, we can consume them directly from those plants or indirectly via meat and, again like vitamins, they are frequently deficient in our modern diets. There are two primary reasons for this: mineral-depleted soil and the refining of food.

Soil gradually loses its mineral content as the plants take up the minerals from the soil, unless the farmer replaces the minerals by adding back mineral-rich manure. However, many of the minerals that pass from plant to us are not needed to make the plant grow, so there is no incentive for the farmer to add them back. Typically, fertilisers only contain nitrogen, phosphate and potassium, so the soils become deficient in the other minerals.

Refining food to make white rice, white flour and white sugar removes up to 90 per cent of some minerals. Foods such as refined breakfast cereals must meet a legal minimum nutrient requirement and therefore have some calcium, iron and B vitamins added back. To help sell them, the packet says 'enriched' or 'with added vitamins and minerals'. This wouldn't be necessary if the food we ate wasn't refined in the first place. Unlike vitamins, minerals are not destroyed by heat when food is cooked, but they do leach into cooking water. Consequently, steaming food conserves mineral content, while boiling does not. If you do boil food, though, you can use the mineral-rich vegetable cooking water as a stock for soups and stews – an effective form of recycling!

The important message here is that getting plenty of these micronutrients in your child's diet won't happen by chance. Vitamin- and mineral-rich fruits, vegetables and wholefoods are unlikely to be their first choice of foods.

## VITAMIN AND MINERAL CHECK

Check your child's intake of vitamins and minerals by answering the questions below.

Does your child...

☐ eat fewer than five servings of fresh fruits and vegetables, excluding potato, every day?

☐ eat fewer than one portion of a dark green vegetable a day?

☐ eat fewer than three portions of fresh or dried tropical fruit a week?

☐ eat seeds or seed oils, such as pumpkin, sunflower or tahini, or unroasted nuts less than three times a week?

☐ typically not take a multivitamin or mineral supplement?

☐ usually eat white bread, rice or pasta instead of brown or wholegrain?

☐ suffer from anxiety, depression or irritability?

☐ suffer from muscle cramps?

☐ have white marks on more than two fingernails?

☐ seem disconnected and find it difficult to relate or communicate?

*If you answer 'yes' to five or more of these questions, the chances are your child isn't getting enough vitamins and minerals.*

## The ultimate headstart

The dividends of giving your child the vitamins and minerals they need right from the start are enormous. That means during pregnancy, and ideally before conception, while breast-feeding and also during the weaning process. Recognition of the importance of good nutrition at this crucial stage in a child's life is behind the UK's Department of Health's Healthy Start scheme, which provides pregnant women and young children from low-income backgrounds with vouchers for fresh fruit and vegetables, and free vitamins.

A 16-year study by the Medical Research Council in the UK shows that optimum nutrition in the early years isn't just critical for your child's physical health; it also affects their intelligence many years later. The research team fed 424 premature babies either a standard or an enriched milk formula containing extra protein, vitamins and minerals. At 18 months, those fed standard milk were doing 'significantly less well' than the others and at eight years old they had IQs up to 14 points lower.[1] Clearly it's important to keep your growing child optimally nourished through pregnancy and early infancy (see chapter 21 for more on this), but remember: it's never too late to increase health-giving vitamins and minerals in your child's diet.

## Nutrients for vitality

Every one of the many essential vitamins and minerals plays a major role in promoting health. Below we list the ones that are most vital to your child's health, along with the symptoms that you might see if your child is deficient in them and the best food families to feed your child to ensure they get enough.

**Vitamin A** is needed for healthy skin, inside and out. It functions as an antioxidant, supporting the immune system, and is crucial for vision. Inadequate intake can result in mouth ulcers, poor night vision, acne, frequent colds and infections, and dry flaky skin. Vitamin A occurs in two main forms: retinol which is found in foods of animal origin, such as liver, meat, cheese and eggs; and beta-carotene, which is found in primarily yellow-orange vegetables, such as carrots, sweet potato and peppers. Beta-carotene is converted into vitamin A in the liver.

**B vitamins** help your child's body make energy out of their food and regulate many bodily processes.

**Vitamin B1 (thiamine)** helps turn glucose, the brain's main fuel, into energy, so one of the first symptoms of thiamine deficiency is mental and physical tiredness. Children low in this vitamin have a poor attention span and concentration.

**Vitamin B2 (riboflavin)** is particularly important for hair, nails and eyes, and if you've ever taken a B-complex or multivitamin and noticed that your pee turned psychedelic yellow, that was the B2! Deficiency symptoms include burning or gritty eyes, sensitivity to bright light, sore tongue, dull or oily hair, eczema, dermatitis, split nails and cracked lips.

**Vitamin B3 (niacin)** is crucial to blood sugar balance and vital in the manufacture of both serotonin (the 'happy' neurotransmitter) and melatonin (the sleep enhancer) from the amino acid tryptophan. This means it's important in keeping your child on an even emotional and mental keel, in good spirits and sleeping well at night. Like all the Bs, it's essential for making energy from food. Deficiency in this vitamin can result in low energy, diarrhoea, insomnia, headaches, depression, irritability and skin conditions such as acne and eczema.

**Vitamin B5 (pantothenic acid)** is your child's key memory and anti-stress vitamin. It is needed to make the memory-boosting neurotransmitter acetylcholine. Signs of deficiency include muscle tremors or cramps, apathy, poor concentration, burning feet or tender heels, nausea, low energy and anxiety or tension.

**Vitamin B6 (pyridoxine)** is needed for hormone production and to make the happy neurotransmitter serotonin. B6 can help relieve stress, and stress also depletes the body's stores of B6. Signs of deficiency include being unable to recall dreams, tingling hands (this can also be a sign of B6 toxicity!), depression, nervousness, irritability, muscle tremors or cramps, low energy or flaky skin.

**Vitamin B12 (cobalamin)** helps the blood carry oxygen and it's needed for DNA synthesis. Vitamin B12 is also essential for nerves. Signs of deficiency include poor hair or skin condition, irritability, anxiety or tension, low energy, constipation, tender or sore muscles and pale skin.

**Folic acid** is essential for brain and nerve function (and their development in pregnancy). It's needed to utilise protein and for red cell formation. Signs of deficiency include anaemia, eczema, cracked lips, anxiety or tension, poor memory or appetite, stomach pains and depression.

This trio, B6, B12 and folic acid, control a critical process in the body called methylation, which is vital in the formation of almost all neurotransmitters. Abnormal methylation lies behind many health problems. These three are also key to managing the levels of an amino acid called homocysteine. Elevated levels of homocysteine have been linked to an increased risk of, among other diseases, cardiovascular problems and osteoporosis.

**Biotin** is particularly important for children as it helps their body use the essential fats to promote healthy skin, hair and nerves. Signs of deficiency include dry skin, poor hair condition, tender or sore muscles, poor appetite or nausea, eczema or dermatitis.

B vitamins are found in a wide variety of foods, especially grains, vegetables and pulses. They are easily destroyed by cooking and processing, and are almost entirely removed in the refining process, so wholegrains, such as oats and barley, and fresh vegetables, such as spinach and watercress, are some of the best sources. Vitamin B12 is the exception here. It's only found in foods of animal origin, such as eggs and fish. Strict vegetarian diets can be almost devoid of B12. If your child is playing host to a healthy population of gut flora, then these bacteria will provide some (see chapter 7 for more on this).

**Vitamin C (ascorbic acid)** is best known for its role in fighting infections, colds and flu. It helps make collagen in the skin, bones and joints, and functions as an antioxidant, protecting against pollution and recycling its fellow antioxidant vitamin E. Like the B vitamins, it helps turn food into energy. Deficiency symptoms include frequent infections or infections that are hard to shift, low energy, easy bruising, bleeding gums and regular nosebleeds. The best place to find vitamin C is in fresh fruits and vegetables, such as broccoli, peppers, kiwis and oranges. Like the B vitamins, it's depleted by light, heat and oxygen, so levels will plummet in food that has been sitting around for a while or that has been heavily processed.

**Vitamin D (cholecalciferol)** is most famous for its role in promoting healthy bones and teeth, because it helps your body take up and utilise calcium. However, in recent years it's been discovered that vitamin D has many other roles within the immune system and is involved in mood, cardiovascular health and cancer protection. Deficiency in this vitamin may be widespread and, unlike the other vitamins, food is not our main source of it. Although vitamin D is a fat-soluble vitamin and is found in some fatty foods, such as oily fish, milk and eggs, you can't get all you need from diet alone. In fact, the reason vitamin D is called the 'sunshine vitamin' is because we make it in our skin in the presence of sunshine. Many people don't get enough sun exposure these days and those particularly at risk of deficiency are dark-skinned people, because the pigment in their skin filters out the UV rays that trigger the production of vitamin D. Children must have regular sun exposure, but of course never to the point of burning. However, many may need a supplement, especially in winter, and supplementation is now routinely recommended for pregnant and breast-feeding women.

**Vitamin E (tocopherol)** is the antioxidant that protects cells and essential fats from damage. It's needed for skin health and the immune system. Signs of deficiency include easy bruising, slow wound-healing, loss of muscle tone and dry skin. Vitamin E is a fat-soluble vitamin and as such is found in oily foods such as seeds, seed oils, nuts, oily fish and wheatgerm.

**Vitamin K (phylloquinone)** is essential for blood-clotting. A deficiency in this vitamin will lead to haemorrhaging. Vitamin K has been routinely given to newborn babies for decades, although this practice has been called into question in recent years. You'll get some Vitamin K in vegetables such as cauliflower, broccoli, cabbage and potatoes, but most of your vitamin K is made for your child by their gut flora. So, the most important thing for this vitamin is that your child has healthy gut flora (see chapter 7 for more on this).

## Mineral marvels

Vitamins get a lot of the good press, but minerals are equally important for your child's growth and development. Let's look at the key players.

**Calcium**, as most people know, is essential for healthy bones and teeth. However, giving children a mineral may be the last thing you'd think of doing to calm them and help them sleep, yet that's also precisely what calcium does, by helping to relax nerve and muscle cells. Signs of deficiency include muscle cramps or tremors, insomnia or nervousness, joint pain and tooth decay. Dairy products provide much of our calcium. However, there are plenty more good sources including almonds, pumpkin seeds, sardines, greens and walnuts.

**Chromium** helps keep blood sugar levels even and reduces sugar cravings. Children deficient in chromium will show signs of poor blood sugar balance, such as mood swings, irritability when they're hungry, sugar cravings and, in more extreme cases, heavy or cold sweats, particularly at night. Chromium is found in wholegrains, but up to 98 per cent of the chromium is removed in the refining process, so a diet featuring plenty of white rice, white pasta and white bread will be deficient in chromium. Other foods that are good for chromium include potatoes, peppers, eggs and chicken.

**Copper** is involved in several key systems in the body. It's needed for collagen, an essential component of skin, blood vessels, bones and joints, and also for proper iron absorption and utilisation, but copper is something of a Jekyll and Hyde mineral, in that an excess of it is also associated with mental health symptoms, such as anxiety and paranoia (see chapter 6 for more on this). Copper deficiency symptoms are rarely seen in children, but shellfish and pulses are the best dietary sources of it.

**Iron** helps the red blood cells transport oxygen around the body and is needed for the body to convert food into energy. Iron deficiency shows up as low energy, fatigue, listlessness and anaemia. The best sources of iron are animal-based foods, such as eggs and meat. Vegetable sources include pumpkin seeds, almonds, pulses and spinach. Vitamin C helps with the absorption of iron, so giving your kids some fresh fruit with their eggs in the morning will increase the iron uptake.

**Magnesium** is typically the second most deficient mineral in children, after zinc. Together with calcium, it's needed in relatively large amounts to form strong bones and teeth. Like calcium, magnesium is also a natural muscle relaxant, aiding sleep and calming hyperactive children. It's essential for energy production, too. Children deficient in magnesium may have difficulty getting to sleep or staying asleep or they may experience restless sleep. They may be anxious, nervous, hyperactive, constipated and have headaches. Muscle cramps, including menstrual cramps, are a clear sign of magnesium deficiency. Green, leafy vegetables are good sources of magnesium and so are nuts and seeds, particularly sesame, sunflower and pumpkin.

**Manganese** helps to form healthy bones and cartilage, tissues and nerves. It activates more than 20 enzymes, which accelerate chemical reactions in the body, helps with blood sugar balance, promotes healthy DNA, is involved in red blood cell production and supports healthy brain function. Signs of deficiency include muscle twitches, 'growing pains', dizziness or a poor sense of balance, fits and convulsions. Tropical fruit such as pineapple and mango are good sources, as are watercress, oats and berries.

**Selenium** is an important antioxidant and it helps to protect against free radicals and carcinogens, as well as supporting the immune system in the fight against infections. A deficiency of selenium in children makes them more susceptible to illness. There is plenty of selenium in seeds and nuts, tuna and mushrooms.

**Zinc** is one of the most critical nutrients for children and the mineral they are most commonly deficient in. Zinc is necessary for growth, immunity and energy production. The average intake in Britain is 7.5mg, which is half the recommended daily allowance (RDA) of 15mg and means that half the British population get less than half the level of zinc thought to protect against deficiency. Children deficient in zinc will probably have white spots on their finger nails or will develop stretch marks if they gain weight quickly. They may also show signs of poor growth, increased susceptibility to infections and a multitude of mental health symptoms, such as hyperactivity, autism, depression, anxiety, anorexia, schizophrenia and delinquency. Zinc also helps children perform in school and there are many times during their development when children need a boost from extra zinc – growth spurts, puberty, stress, infections, excess copper, blood sugar problems and even an inherited need for more of this mineral. Boys need extra zinc from about age 12, as zinc is required for sperm production. However, any 'seed' food – nuts, seeds and the germ of grains – provides zinc, and meat and fish are rich sources, but none is richer than oysters, as a single oyster can contain as much as 15mg of zinc!

As you can see, if children eat a varied diet of fresh foods and wholefoods they will consume the best range and quantity of all these wonderful nutrients (see part 4 for more on improving your child's diet and supplements).

## Antioxidants – protecting your child

We live in a highly polluted world and there may be little you can do to avoid many of the pollutants, but you can protect your child from some of this pollution from the inside, with antioxidants.

Antioxidants are the antidote to oxidants, also known as 'free radicals', which are highly unstable molecules that can trigger cellular damage. They are a byproduct of normal body processes and of combustion. In the body, oxidants are produced every time glucose is 'burnt' within a cell to make energy and they can go on to damage the essential fats, proteins and phospholipids that make up your child's brain and body. In the environment, they can result from, say, a car burning petrol as fuel. If we see oxidants as the sparks from something burning, such as food frying or a smoking cigarette, antioxidants are like fire-proof gloves that prevent the sparks from damaging your cells.

A single puff of a cigarette contains a trillion oxidants, which rapidly travel into the brain. This is why smoking around children is especially bad news. Less avoidable are the oxidants from exhaust fumes, particularly diesel. These have an insidious effect on your child's body and brain, and that's why it's crucial for your child to have a good intake of antioxidants.

There are many members of this fire-fighting team and they work together to protect your child. To give your child maximum protection, it's worth making sure their daily supplement contains them, as well as giving them antioxidant-rich foods.

## Food sources of the main antioxidants

- **Beta-carotene** – carrots, sweet potatoes, dried apricots (soaked first), squash and watercress

- **Vitamin C** – broccoli, peppers, kiwi fruit, berries, tomatoes and citrus fruit

- **Vitamin E** – seeds and their cold-pressed oils, wheatgerm, nuts, beans and fish

- **Selenium** – oysters, Brazil nuts, seeds, molasses, tuna and mushrooms

- **Glutathione** – tuna, pulses, nuts, seeds, garlic and onions

- **Anthocyanidins** – berries, cherries, red grapes, beetroot and prunes

- **Lipoic acid** – red meat, potatoes, carrots, yams, beetroot and spinach

- **Coenzyme Q** – sardines, mackerel, nuts and seeds.

Of course, it's also about what your child doesn't eat. As well as the oxidants we all make just from burning glucose as fuel, eating a piece of crispy meat introduces millions of these bad guys, so it's important not to overcook, burn or char food. A barbecue is great fun, but do cook on lower flames and ensure your children's sausages are gently browned and cooked all the way through, not charred black on the outside. If you like to fry food, try sautéing it gently on a low heat with the lid on the pan. If the oil spits or smokes in the frying pan, it's too hot.

## Summary

To ensure your child gets plenty of vitamins and minerals:

- Make sure your child eats foods rich in antioxidants – fruits, vegetables, seeds and fish. Their diet should include at least five, and ideally seven, servings of fresh fruit and vegetables a day.

- Serve nuts and seeds daily, and choose wholefoods, such as wholegrains, lentils, beans and brown rice, rather than refined food.

- Give your child an 'optimum nutrition' multivitamin and mineral every day (see chapter 25 for more on this).

- Don't smoke and avoid charring or crisping food to avoid overexposure to oxidants.

# Chapter 6

·

# Anti-nutrients and how to avoid them

Eating plenty of the good stuff is only half the story. It's equally important, as we saw with fats, to keep your kids away from the bad stuff. We call this bad stuff, collectively, anti-nutrients. An anti-nutrient is any substance that depletes the body of nutrients or interferes with the nutrient's metabolism. Trans fats, oxidants and sugar are anti-nutrients, as we've seen. Now let's look at the rest of the nasties – toxic minerals, additives and preservatives.

In the last chapter we looked at some of the minerals essential for your child's health, but not all minerals are good news. Some, such as the 'heavy metals' lead and mercury, are thoroughly bad news, particularly for your child's brain and nervous system. For example, a high intake of mercury can have a disastrous effect on intelligence and behaviour in children and adults alike.

### CASE HISTORY *Anthony, age nine*

Anthony had been diagnosed with dysgraphia, a learning difficulty that specifically affects handwriting. Before bringing him to us, his parents had already noticed that his writing was directly affected by sugar and E-numbers, and they had taken these out of his diet, to good effect. We conducted a hair analysis which showed that he had high levels of the toxic metal mercury in his hair. We increased his intake of zinc, selenium and vitamin C to help his body remove the mercury and three months later Anthony and his mother were happy to report that his handwriting had improved significantly.

## Heavy metals – the usual suspects

You might think you'd only be exposed to heavy metals if you lived or worked near a toxic dumping ground, but in fact they are shockingly common in the environment.

### Cadmium – peril as you puff

Cigarette smoke is laden with cadmium, a heavy metal associated with disturbed mental performance and increased aggression. This nasty also lurks in car exhaust fumes and there can be small amounts in food, especially if it's refined, because beneficial minerals that act as cadmium protectors, such as selenium and zinc, are taken out during the refining process. Cadmium also knocks out zinc, so passive smokers will need more.

Keep your children away from cigarette smoke. If you smoke, quit – this is the best way to prevent your children from picking up the habit, while protecting them from heavy metal contamination.

### Aluminium – toxic takeaway

Aluminium is found in a staggering array of modern products. Aluminium trays and foils are widely used as food packaging by supermarkets, fast-food outlets and other food-handling operations, and the stuff also turns up in many common household products. It's in antacids, some processed cheeses, toothpaste tubes, anti-perspirants, pots and pans, even our water.

Not all aluminium will enter the body, however. For example, aluminium will leach from a pan only under certain circumstances, but if old-fashioned aluminium cookware is used to heat something acidic like tea, tomatoes or rhubarb, it will leach particles of aluminium into the water. Also, the more zinc-deficient you are, the more aluminium you absorb. To be safe, it's best not to grill food directly on aluminium foil. Instead, use the grill shelf and place the foil underneath the shelf. Adequate Vitamin C helps the body handle aluminium.

## Mercury – why hatters were mad

The phrase 'mad as a hatter' originated in the 18th and 19th centuries, when mercury compounds were used to make felt for hats. When the felt was boiled, then steamed into shape, the hatmakers absorbed the mercury-laden fumes. Mercury can cause depression, irritability, loss of coordination and other distressing symptoms, and the hatmakers' 'madness' was all down to the way the mercury had disturbed their brain processes.

Mercury is, in fact, very toxic indeed. Small amounts reach us from contaminated foods, pharmaceuticals, cosmetics and amalgam tooth fillings, and it has also been used as a constituent of thimerosal, found in diptheria and hepatitis vaccines, although this practice has recently been stopped. Mercury is also present in low-energy light bulbs and mercury thermometers, and so care must be taken when disposing of breakages.

Of particular concern, however, is fish caught in polluted waters. Mercury is used in a number of chemical processes, and accidents and illegal dumping have resulted in a rise in mercury levels in some areas, including the English Channel. Fish, especially larger fish like tuna, swordfish, marlin and shark, store the mercury and we end up ingesting it if we eat them.

The problem is that oily fish such as tuna are a valuable source of omega-3 essential fats. The chart below lists coldwater fish in terms of the inverse ratio of omega-3s to mercury, with the best having the greatest amount of omega-3 to the lowest amount of mercury. There may be significantly lower amounts of omega-3 in farmed salmon compared to wild salmon, because the quantity of essential fat in the fish depends to a large extent on the quality of its diet.

**INVERSE RATIO OF OMEGA-3S TO MERCURY IN COLDWATER FISH**

|  | Omega-3 g/100g | Mercury mg/kg | Omega-3/ mercury |
| --- | --- | --- | --- |
| Fresh wild salmon | 2.7 | 0.05 | 54.0 |
| Canned sardines | 1.57 | 0.04 | 39.3 |
| Canned and smoked salmon | 1.54 | 0.04 | 38.5 |
| Fresh mackerel | 1.93 | 0.06 | 35.1 |
| Herring (kipper) | 1.31 | 0.04 | 32.8 |
| Trout | 1.15 | 0.06 | 19.2 |
| Fresh tuna | 1.5 | 0.4 | 3.8 |
| Cod | 0.25 | 0.11 | 2.3 |
| Fresh sole | 0.1 | 0.05 | 2.0 |
| Canned tuna | 0.37 | 0.19 | 1.9 |
| Marlin (? = guestimate) | ?2 | 1.1 | 1.8 |
| Swordfish (? = guestimate) | ?2 | 1.4 | 1.4 |

## The copper controversy

Copper is both an essential mineral and a toxic one. It's rare to be deficient in copper, unless your diet is very high in refined foods, but copper water pipes do leach small amounts of copper into water and, if you live in a soft-water area or in a house with new copper piping that hasn't yet become calcified, your family can be exposed to toxic levels of copper. Zinc helps the body get rid of any excess copper, but if your child is zinc-deficient, they may not be able to do this.

## Lead – trouble in mind

In the 1990s there were a number of important studies that showed consistently lower IQ in children whose blood, hair or baby teeth contained the highest levels of lead. When Herbert Needleman, an associate professor of child psychiatry at the School of Medicine, University of Pittsburgh, conducted a follow-up study of children who had had elevated lead levels 11 years earlier, he found a sevenfold increase in the odds of those children failing to graduate from high school. They also had a lower class standing, higher levels of absenteeism and were more likely to have reading disabilities, and poor vocabulary, motor skills, reaction time and hand–eye coordination.[1]

Fortunately, since the advent of unleaded petrol, lead should be much less of a problem these days. Or so we thought, until 2007, when there were record numbers of product recalls for toys manufactured in China, the majority of which were related to excess lead levels in the paint. These included products from well known brands such as Fisher-Price, Thomas and Friends, and Barbie. Hopefully, as a result of this staggering array of recalls, there will be more stringent checks made on imported toys in future to ensure that our children are not exposed to lead.

Some lead remains in the environment, but the most likely source these days is drinking water from old lead pipes. Symptoms of lead toxicity include lowered IQ, aggression and headaches.

## How to handle the heavies

A high intake of heavy metals in children has been associated with mood swings, poor impulse control and aggressive behaviour, poor attention span, depression and apathy, disturbed sleep patterns, and impaired memory and intellectual performance. If your child has symptoms like these, we recommend you have them tested for heavy metals.

## Hair mineral analysis – the heavy metal MOT

There's a simple way to find out if these heavy and toxic minerals could be affecting your child – a hair mineral analysis. By analysing a small amount of hair, your child can be effectively screened not only for the bad guys, such as cadmium, aluminium, mercury and lead, but also for the good guys, such as magnesium, zinc, chromium, manganese and so on. At around £50, it's well worth it.

However, what do you do if your child has raised levels of toxic minerals? Luckily, many essential minerals have an antagonistic relationship with heavy metals. This means that taking more of the essential minerals depletes the toxic ones, so once you've done a hair analysis you should see a nutritional therapist for tailored advice to gently detox your child (see Resources).

## Foods that fight heavy metals

Meanwhile, you can certainly improve your child's detoxification, if they need it, by following the general nutrition guidelines in this book, ensuring they get plenty of antioxidants from fresh fruits and vegetables, fibre from pulses, wholegrains and vegetables, and also plenty of water.

In terms of specific foods, there are a few that can help keep your child's system 'clean'. Garlic, onions and eggs contain sulphur-rich amino acids, specifically methionine and cystine, which protect against cadmium, mercury and lead toxicity. Pectin in apples, carrots and citrus fruits also helps to remove heavy metals – yet another reason for an apple a day!

## Keeping your child chemical free

In the last 50 years alone, some 3,500 new chemicals have been added to food, with over 200,000 tonnes of these chemical additives being put into our food each year – approximately 4.5kg per person. In all, the European Union sanctions 395 additives: 71 thickeners and emulsifiers, 64 colours, 54 preservatives, 54 antioxidants, 54 anti-caking agents and acidity regulators, 52 miscellaneous, 27 additional chemicals and 19 flavour enhancers. Up to 4.5l of pesticides and herbicides may have been sprayed on and around the fruit and vegetables consumed by the average person in a year. Meanwhile, a further 3,000 chemicals have been introduced into our homes.[2] Some of our children, indeed perhaps all of us, aren't coping well with this chemical onslaught.

The absolute safety of many of these compounds is questionable. Industry is required to provide some safety data on individual chemicals, but there is no data whatsoever on the effect of all (or any combination) of these on an individual. Most of these compounds can be classed as anti-nutrients – substances that interfere with our ability to absorb or use essential nutrients, or, in some cases, that promote the loss of essential nutrients from the body.

A high intake of anti-nutrient chemicals has been associated with asthma, eczema, dermatitis, mood swings, poor impulse control and aggressive behaviour, poor attention span, depression and apathy, disturbed sleep patterns, and impaired memory and intellectual performance. The best way to remedy or indeed prevent these kinds of symptoms is to keep these chemicals out of your child's life as much as possible.

## Battling the additive blues

In 2004, the UK's Food Standards Agency (FSA) commissioned a research team at the University of Southampton to investigate the effect of a range of additives and a preservative on the behaviour of 1,873 three-year-old children. They found that the children's behaviour was worse when the food colourings – a mixture of sunset yellow (E110), tartrazine (E102), carmoisine (E122) and ponceau 4R (E124) – and the preservative (sodium benzoate) were in their diet than when they weren't. Interestingly, the effect was no different for children who were previously diagnosed hyperactive, compared with those who were not.[3]

The FSA took no action based on these results. Instead, it commissioned a similar study on 153 three-year-old and 144 eight- and nine-year-old children who were not hyperactive. They tested the same additives and preservative as above, with the addition of the colour allura red (E129). The results were strikingly similar, with signs of hyperactivity seen in all the children.[4] The FSA says that unless substances such as additives and preservatives are proved to be 'a danger to human health' it doesn't have the power to ban them, so it's down to parents to scrutinise labels if they want to avoid additives in their children's diets.

Dr Neil Ward from the University of Surrey decided to test what happened to minerals when drinks containing tartrazine, which is still added to many popular soft drinks for children to colour it yellowy orange, were consumed. He gave children drinks which looked and tasted identical, but some contained tartrazine and some didn't. He found that adding tartrazine to drinks increased the amount of zinc excreted in the urine, perhaps because the tartrazine bound to zinc in the blood and prevented it from being used by the body.[5]

In this study, like many others, Ward also found emotional and behavioural changes in every child who consumed tartrazine. Four out of the ten children in the study had severe reactions, three experiencing an outbreak of eczema or having an asthma attack within 45 minutes of ingestion. Tartrazine is one of the first of over 1,000 chemical food additives that has been proven to be an anti-nutrient.

The primary reasons for adding chemicals to food is to make the food look better by changing its colour, and to preserve and stabilise it. Most of the additives are synthetic compounds, some with known negative health effects. But more importantly, we don't know what the long-term consequences of consuming such large amounts of additives are. This is especially true for children whose brains and bodies are still developing. It is therefore best to avoid all additives, with a few notable exceptions.

**Acceptable additives**

- The colours E101(vitamin B2) and E160 (carotene, vitamin A)

- The antioxidants E300–304 (vitamin C) and E306–309 (tocopherols, such as vitamin E)

- The emulsifier E322 (lecithin)

- The stabilisers E375 (niacin) and E440 (pectin).

## Unacceptable additives

The chart below gives the most up-to-date information on the worst food additives, but remember that you won't just find these additives in food as many medications that are formulated for children, such as cough syrups, contain colours, too. In general, there is a distinct lack of research on the negative effects of food additives, because food manufacturers have no desire to carry out studies beyond the minimum requirements to enable them to continue to put these additives into food.

### TOP 20 ADDITIVES TO AVOID

#### Allura red AC  •  (E129)

*How it's used:* As a colouring in snacks, sauces, preserves, soups, wine and cider.

*What you need to know:* Avoid if your child has asthma, rhinitis (including hay fever) or urticaria (an allergic rash also known as hives).

#### Amaranth  •  (E123)

*How it's used:* As a colouring in jams, jellies and cake decorations.

*What you need to know:* Avoid if your child has asthma, rhinitis, urticaria or other allergies. It's banned in the US.

### Aspartame • (E951)

*How it's used:* As a sweetener in snacks, sweets, desserts and 'diet' foods.

*What you need to know:* Recent reports show long-term, high-dose use may cause headaches, blindness and seizures. May affect people with the genetic disorder phenylketonuria (PKU).

### Benzoic acid • (E210)

*How it's used:* As a preservative in many foods, including drinks, low-sugar products, cereals and meat products.

*What you need to know:* Can temporarily inhibit the function of digestive enzymes and may deplete glycine levels. Avoid if your child has asthma, rhinitis, urticaria or other allergies.

### Brilliant black BN • (E151)

*How it's used:* As a colouring in drinks, sauces, snacks and cheese.

*What you need to know:* Avoid if your child has asthma, rhinitis, urticaria or other allergies.

### Butylated hydroxy-anisole (BHA) • (E320)

*How it's used:* As a preservative, particularly in fat-containing foods, confectionery and meats.

*What you need to know:* The International Agency for Research on Cancer say that BHA is possibly carcinogenic to humans. BHA also interacts with nitrites to form chemicals known to cause changes in the DNA of cells.

### Calcium/potassium benzoate • (E213/E212)

*How it's used:* As a preservative in many foods, including drinks, low-sugar products, cereals and meat products.

*What you need to know:* Can temporarily inhibit the function of digestive enzymes and may deplete levels of the amino acid glycine. Avoid if your child has asthma, rhinitis, or urticaria.

### Calcium sulphite  •  (E226)

*How it's used:* As a preservative in a vast array of foods, including burgers, biscuits and frozen mushrooms.

*What you need to know:* Sulphites are banned from many foods in the US, because they make old produce look fresh. They can cause bronchial problems, flushing or reddening of the skin, low blood pressure, tingling and anaphylactic shock. The International Labour Organisation (ILO) says avoid them if you suffer from bronchial asthma, cardiovascular or respiratory problems, or emphysema.

---

### Monosodium glutamate (MSG)  •  (E621)

*How it's used:* As a flavour enhancer.

*What you need to know:* Those sensitive to MSG experience pressure on the head, tightness of the face, burning sensations, headache, nausea, chest pains and seizures. Many baby-food producers have stopped adding MSG to their products.

---

### Ponceau 4R, Cochineal red A  •  (E124)

*How it's used:* As a colouring.

*What you need to know:* Those who suffer from asthma, rhinitis or urticaria may find their symptoms become worse after consumption.

---

### Sodium benzoate  •  (E211)

*How it's used:* As a preservative.

*What you need to know:* Recent evidence suggests it causes hyperactivity in children and may promote oxidative damage.

---

### Potassium nitrate  •  (E249)

*How it's used:* As a preservative in cured meats and canned meat products.

*What you need to know:* It can lower the oxygen-carrying capacity of the blood; it may combine with other substances to form nitrosamines, which are carcinogenic; and it may have an atrophying effect on the adrenal gland.

---

### Propyl p-hydroxy-benzoate, propyl-paraben, paraben • (E216)

*How it's used:* As a preservative in cereals, snacks, paté, meat products and confectionery.

*What you need to know:* Parabens have frequently been identified as the cause of chronic dermatitis.

---

### Saccharin and its Na, K and Ca salts • (E954)

*How it's used:* As a sweetener in diet and no-added-sugar products.

*What you need to know:* The International Agency for Research on Cancer has concluded that saccharin is possibly carcinogenic to humans.

---

### Sodium metabisulphite • (E223)

*How it's used:* Widely used as a preservative and antioxidant.

*What you need to know:* May provoke life-threatening asthma – a woman developed severe asthma after eating a salad with a vinegar-based dressing containing E223.

---

### Sodium sulphite • (E221)

*How it's used:* as a preservative in wine and other processed foods.

*What you need to know:* Sulphites have been associated with triggering asthma attacks. Most asthmatics are sensitive to sulphites in food.

---

### Stannous chloride (tin) • (E512)

*How it's used:* As an antioxidant and colour-retention agent in canned and bottled foods and fruit juices.

*What you need to know:* Acute poisoning – nausea, vomiting, diarrhoea and headaches – has been reported from ingestion of fruit juices containing concentrations of tin greater than 250mg/l.

---

### Sulphur dioxide • (E220)

*How it's used:* As a preservative.

*What you need to know:* Sulphur dioxide reacts with a wide range of substances found in food, including various essential vitamins, minerals, enzymes and essential fats. The most common adverse reaction to sulphites is bronchial problems, particularly in those prone to asthma. Other adverse reactions may include hypotension (low blood pressure), flushing, tingling sensations and anaphylactic shock. The ILO says you should avoid E220 if you suffer from conjunctivitis, bronchitis, bronchial asthma, cardiovascular disease or emphysema.

### Sunset yellow FCF, Orange/yellow • (SE110)

*How it's used:* As a colouring.

*What you need to know:* Some animal studies have indicated growth retardation and severe weight loss related to this additive. Avoid if your child has asthma, rhinitis or urticaria.

### Tartrazine • (E102)

*How it's used:* As a colouring.

*What you need to know:* May cause allergic reactions in perhaps 15 per cent of the population. May cause asthmatic attacks and has been implicated in bouts of hyperactivity disorder in children. Those who suffer from asthma, rhinitis or urticaria may find their symptoms become worse after consumption.

*Source: P. Cox and P. Brusseau,* Secret Ingredients (Bantam, 1997), *with permission of Peter Cox and Bantam Books*

# Go for organic foods

The presence of pesticide residue, particularly on fruits and vegetables, is a widely acknowledged and regularly reported fact. Again, due to the paucity of research, it's difficult to say how significant the impact on your child's health might be of a single pesticide and it's impossible to know the effect of a cocktail of these chemicals.

The best way to avoid pesticides is to give organic produce to your child whenever you can. Of course, organic food also contains higher amounts of health-giving nutrients because the soil is naturally enriched. Organic food is often perceived as being much more expensive than conventionally grown food, but in some cases there is little difference in price, so do what you can within your budget. In addition, most organic food hasn't been forced to grow fast and so it contains less water. This means three organic carrots will fill you up as much as four regular supermarket carrots, so even if the price is 25 per cent more, at the end of the day you're getting just as much carrot, plus all the extra nutrients and no pesticide or herbicide residues, which amounts to good value for money.

However, is it better to eat organic apples that have been flown half-way around the world or conventionally grown local apples that have not travelled so far? This is quite a conundrum, but by buying fruits and vegetables that are in season you are more likely to be able to get food that is both local and organic. In the UK, that means apples and pears in winter, blackberries and plums in summer, for example. Also, go for whole lettuces rather than 'bagged' salads since these are less likely to be chemically treated to maintain 'freshness'.

Organic means much more than 'pesticide free', though. Organic meat or fish has to adhere to strict rules, not only in terms of what the animals are fed, but also in relation to how they are reared and the use of any growth hormones or antibiotics. As a result, it's well worth paying the extra for organic meat, eggs, farmed fish and milk.

## Summary

To help keep your child free from anti-nutrients:

- Give a multivitamin and mineral supplement that includes zinc, selenium and vitamin C for toxic mineral protection (see chapter 25 for more on this).

continues →

- Have a hair mineral analysis done for your child, available through nutritional therapists (see Resources).

- Read labels and avoid foods containing chemical food additives.

- Stick to whole, natural foods as much as possible, since these should be additive-free, although you will still need to check labels.

- Choose organic food, including meat, eggs, milk, fish, and fruit and vegetables.

- Cut down on chemical use in the home by using natural cleaning products and avoiding unnecessary room and fabric 'deodorisers'.

# Chapter 7

·

# Getting to the gut of the matter

You've heard the old adage 'you are what you eat' and, as we've discussed in previous chapters, it's certainly true that your child is literally constructed from the food that he or she eats. In actual fact, it's more accurate to say that 'you are what you eat, digest and absorb'. It's one thing to eat the food, but how do the nutrients become available to the body, so that they can be used in the building and repair process? This is where the digestive system comes in.

You can think of the digestive system as a long tube that runs from one end of the body to the other – from mouth to anus or from chew to poo. Its job is to take the food that we put in at the mouth end and break it down into its component parts, namely the nutrients we've been talking about – amino acids, fatty acids, simple sugars, vitamins, minerals and so on.

First, the food is broken down by the action of chewing in the mouth while simultaneously being swished around with saliva that contains enzymes. These are natural chemicals that help to break the food down into smaller molecules.

Next the food enters the stomach, where more enzymes and stomach acid continue the process of breaking it down. From here,

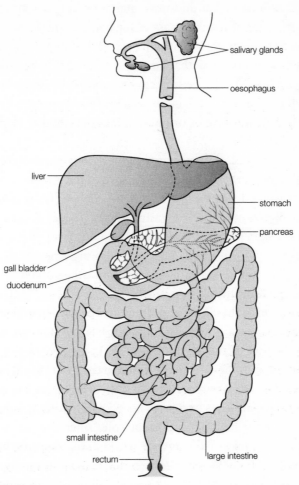

*The digestive system*

the food, which now has a soupy consistency, enters the first part of the intestines, where yet more enzymes, contained in the 'digestive juices' from the pancreas and gall bladder, get to work to continue the process of breaking the food down into its smallest constituent parts – nutrients.

Then the absorption of these nutrients into the body from the tube we call the gut begins. The 'gut wall' is a very thin membrane

– it's just a single cell in thickness, making it only 0.03mm thick or about one third of the thickness of the paper in this book. The gut wall needs to allow these nutrients across, but it also acts as a barrier, so that 'bits of food' that have not yet been fully broken down can't get across. Under certain circumstances the integrity of the gut wall can be lost, allowing undigested food into the body and resulting in food allergies or intolerances (see chapter 13 for more on this).

This process of absorption continues along a good portion of the gut's considerable length. Then, once all the goodness has been taken from the food, the gut's function changes from transportation and digestion of food to waste removal. In fact, it's not just the 'leftovers', such as indigestible fibre from our food, that continues along the gut at this point. The body also uses the gut as a waste conveyor, dumping waste resulting from other bodily processes into the gut for removal from the body.

In addition to these two important jobs of getting nutrients into the body and getting waste out, the gut has another vital function as a major part of the immune system. In fact, 70–80 per cent of your child's immune system is located in their gut. You'll be aware that the immune system is the body's defence system; it attacks foreign invaders and does its best to keep us free from disease. In the gut it has a particularly important role, since the gut regularly receives big chunks of the outside world in the shape of food that is teeming with the bacteria, viruses and fungi that surround us in the air. We are protected from these critters on the outside by our skin and its many defence mechanisms – our nasal and oral passages, for example, use various secretions, hairs, coughing and sneezing to protect us from invasion. In the gut, a special environment exists to protect us from this on-going invasion. Key to this special environment is our gut bacteria. The human gut plays host to a staggering $10^{14}$ (100,000,000,000,000) indigenous bacteria. This is approximately 10–100 times greater than the total number of cells in the human body. What's more, there are over 2,000 different species of bacteria![1]

As we mentioned, the immune system in the gut has an important role in reacting to and mounting a defence against foreign invaders. However, it has an even more important immune function in that it must not react unnecessarily. The immune system must discern friend (that is, your child's food) from foe (for example, a harmful virus or bacterium). This 'not reacting' is called tolerance, or more specifically mucosal tolerance, since the gut wall is known as a mucous membrane. Mucosal tolerance is one of the hottest areas of immunology research today. One of the major players in the mucosal tolerance game is an antibody called Secretory IgA or SIgA for short. It is in constant conversation with the immune system, reassuring it that the molecules passing through are food and that all is well. Without this constant reassurance from SIgA, the immune system turns into a nervous soldier firing at everything that moves.

So how do you know when your child's gut is working well, delivering nutrients into the body, transporting waste out and maintaining an appropriate immune response? A good digestive system is free from symptoms and produces one to three well-formed, mid-brown, soft and not excessively malodorous stools daily.

## DIGESTION CHECK

Check your child's digestive system by answering the questions below.

Does your child...

☐  have less than one bowel movement daily?

☐  have to strain to have a bowel movement?

☐  have excessively smelly stools?

☐  have excessive or smelly wind?

☐  have frequent 'tummy aches' or indigestion?

continues →

☐ have diarrhoea or loose stools regularly?

☐ have immune-related health problems such as frequent infections?

☐ have inflammatory health problems such as eczema or asthma?

☐ have a history of two or more courses of antibiotics per five years of life?

☐ have a pot belly and/or puffy eyes or face?

*If you answer 'yes' to five or more of these questions, the chances are your child's digestive system is not working well.*

## Good digestion starts with chewing

Good digestion starts in the mouth. Thorough chewing of food is essential. It not only physically breaks the food into smaller pieces, but it also ensures that the saliva, with its digesting enzymes, gets well mixed in to begin the chemical digestion of the food. If meal-times are rushed or food is eaten on the run, poor chewing habits can easily develop. Try to instil good chewing habits in your children from the start, setting a good example yourself. You can suggest that every mouthful is chewed around 30 times or have them feel the texture of the food with their tongue before they swallow it. There shouldn't be any lumps. If it's impossible to avoid a rushed breakfast in your household, a breakfast of porridge with ground seeds and grated apple, which involves minimal chewing, would be a better option than a heavy muesli.

Digestion in the stomach relies on the production of sufficient stomach acid and an enzyme called pepsin. Like all substances produced by the body, nutrients are required. Of particular importance for stomach acid production is zinc. This mineral is in great demand in children, because it's required for growth and is often deficient in the diet. Also important to get stomach acid flowing is the anticipation of eating! A pause for breath (or several breaths) before tucking into a meal really improves digestibility. Low stomach acid can cause indigestion and reflux as food sits in the stomach for an extended period. This may be mistaken for excess stomach acid as the symptoms appear similar. Before you reach for the antacids, try getting your child to really chew thoroughly and eat slowly, pausing for a few calming breaths before eating and throughout the meal if need be.

## Bacterial balance

As we saw above, a good balance of gut flora is essential for healthy digestion. The gut of a newborn has long been thought to be entirely sterile, although emerging evidence suggests that this may not be the case. The bacteria that do inhabit your child's gut, though, arrived there when they made their way through the birth canal, from the air around them as they took their first breaths, and from the skin and clothing of those who held them. This apparently random selection of bacteria then evolves into a mix that is unique to your child. The bacteria live off the food that your child eats and off the debris of the constantly shedding cells of the gut wall, which is renewed about every four days.

If your child has antibiotics, these indiscriminately obliterate the bacterial population of their gut, destroying the delicate balance and leaving only those species resistant to the antibiotic to proliferate. This entirely alters the 'breeding stock'. Antibiotics are prescribed much less readily these days and should only be given for an identified bacterial infection. However, if your child must take antibiotics, they should certainly be followed by some probiotics, which are a supplemental form of good bacteria. A good probiotic will provide the bacteria species lactobacillus acidophillus and bifidobacter to repopulate the gut. Don't use the heavily marketed probiotic mini drinks. These are generally very high in sugar and are not good value for money. Natural yoghurt is a good source of some species of lactobacillus and these will exert a good influence as they pass along the digestive tract. However, unlike a good probiotic supplement, they won't take up residence, so continued use is necessary for benefit. Another useful supplement is saccharomyces boulardii, although as a yeast this is not technically a probiotic. It stimulates the gut to produce SIgA, the important immune player that supports tolerance in the gut and also makes the environment of the gut more hospitable to the probiotics, encouraging them to take up residence. Saccharomyces boulardii is generally well tolerated even in people with a yeast intolerance, but since it can aggravate eczema in sensitive individuals a graded introduction is recommended.

## Fabulous fibre

Also important for the health of your child's digestive system is the quality of their food. Like all bodily systems, the digestive system needs a constant supply of nutrients for its growth and repair. Indigestible fibre, while not technically a nutrient, is required in good quantities in the diet for several reasons. Firstly, it's fermented by the gut flora for food. Secondly, this fermentation process produces nutrients for their host, such as the B vitamins and vitamin K. Thirdly, fibre is necessary to help the food move along the length of the gut. The gut moves food along through a series of squeezing movements called peristalsis, but without enough fibre there isn't enough bulk to squeeze against. Finally, fibre has a spongy property that enables it to hold water. This keeps stools soft and makes them easy to pass. Adequate fibre, from vegetables, pulses and oats in the diet, not only eases constipation, it can also help children whose stools tend to be loose too. Fibre supplements such as psyllium seeds husks or ground linseeds, both taken with plenty of water, are a gentle way of providing bulk to the stool. Wheat bran fibre can be irritating to the gut for many children.

Not surprisingly, plenty of water in the diet helps the gut function properly, too. As we mentioned above, the food that leaves the stomach has a soupy consistency. As this food journeys along the digestive tract, the water is absorbed from it into the body. If water is in short supply, the stools that form at the far end of the gut will become harder and harder to pass, resulting in constipation. Once a child has had the painful experience of passing hard stools, they may develop an aversion to passing stools at all. This 'failing to heed the call' makes the problem worse, as the longer stools remain in the colon, the drier and harder they become.

## Good digestion is vital for your child's health

Follow the recommendations above to optimise your child's digestion, but if your child continues to have regular constipation, diarrhoea, bloating or tummy aches, take them to see your GP and a suitably qualified nutritional therapist. Don't accept, 'It's just toddler diarrhoea and they'll grow out of it.' Gut health provides the foundations to your child's overall long-term health and, in our many years of experience, it is the child that has these digestive symptoms as a youngster who goes on to be plagued with persistent ear, nose and throat infections and lowered immunity throughout childhood and into adulthood.

### Summary

To ensure your child's digestive system is working well:

- Choose a wholefood diet which provides plenty of fibre to keep your child's friendly flora well fed, and avoid refined foods.

- Encourage thorough chewing of food and avoid rushed mealtimes.

continues →

- Antibiotics should only be used if absolutely necessary. If repeated infections are an issue for your child, look to the source (see chapter 14 for more on this).

- A good probiotic and saccharomyces boulardii should be used to help restore bacterial balance in the gut, particularly following antibiotic treatment (see Products and supplements directory).

# PART 2

·

# GIVE YOUR CHILD A HEAD START

As you've discovered, the right food underpins your child's health. Furthermore, food directly affects how your child thinks and feels because their brains (and yours) are made of it. Eating the best foods has been proven to boost IQ, improve mood and behaviour, hone memory and concentration, and sharpen reading and writing skills. In this part of the book you'll discover how to maximise your child's potential for educational performance, while helping them to enjoy life and feel personally fulfilled.

# Chapter 8

# Feeding your child's brain

Are your child's mind and memory sharp? Can they concentrate and stay alert for an hour? Is their mood stable? Do they sleep well, get to sleep easily, and wake up fizzing with energy and raring to go? Or are they often exhausted, easily distracted and prone to overreact, or get upset or angry easily?

Now you've learnt the basics about the nutrients your child needs for optimum nutrition, it's time to focus on what your child's intelligence is all about. As you'll see in this book, study after study shows that you can increase intelligence, attention span, concentration, problem-solving ability, emotional response, mood and physical coordination – all the facets of intelligence – simply by changing what goes into and on to their bowls, plates and lunch boxes.

## Food for the brain

In 2005, we founded a charity to promote the link between nutrition and mental health. The charity, Food for the Brain, conducted a survey of over 10,000 children in Britain, comparing food intake with academic performance, behaviour and health. The children were of all ages, with three-quarters of them aged between six and 15 years old. The survey, the largest ever in Britain, found that more than one in three children in the survey had problems behaving and performing academically, and there was a strong association between poor eating habits, poor behaviour and academic performance. A number of key foods were identified as having a substantially beneficial effect on both behaviour and academic performance.

Some key findings of the survey were:

- Children who eat diets high in fried food, takeaways or foods cooked in hot fat are three times more likely to be badly behaved.

- Children who eat vegetables, oily fish, nuts and seeds do best at school.

- Children on the best diets have 11 per cent higher academic scores than those on the worst diets.

- The best foods for behaviour are fruit and vegetables. Those children eating the most of both are twice as likely to be well behaved.

- The worst foods are fried, takeaway and processed food, ready meals and sugar.

- A massive 44 per cent of children who eat this type of junk food most days suffer from bad behaviour, compared with only 16 per cent of children who never eat fried or takeaway food.

- Children who ate nuts and seeds daily did twice as well academically as children who didn't eat nuts and seeds at all.

- The best foods for good academic scores are dark green leafy vegetables, oily fish and water. The worst foods are processed foods and ready meals.

The survey was published in September 2007 and is available at www.foodforthebrain.org. The Food for the Brain website provides all sorts of useful information for parents and schools, and you can also complete the survey questionnaire to identify where your child could be eating better food for the brain.

While the practical advice we give you is based on solid scientific research, we feel even more confident about our conclusions because we have worked with hundreds of children over the past two decades. Some of them were disabled, some coping with serious behavioural problems, yet all were transformed once their own unique optimum nutrition needs were discovered and fulfilled.

Every day at the Brain Bio Centre clinic, part of the Food for the Brain charity, we see children who are struggling to learn, develop and adapt. Our job as nutritional therapists who specialise in children's development is not only to find out what's wrong – be it a food allergy, a chemical sensitivity or a nutrient deficiency – but also to show parents how to make good food that children like, wean them off sugar and expand the range of healthy foods on the daily menu (see part 4 for more on this).

As well as working one to one with kids and parents at the Brain Bio Centre, we've tested our theories in primary schools, secondary schools and special educational needs schools, through the work of the Food for the Brain Schools Project, again with staggering improvements in learning and behaviour.

Much of our work has been with children and young adults diagnosed with ADHD, autism, Asperger's, depression and even psychosis. The usual routes for children with these conditions are prescription drugs or specialised psychological support. We believe that optimum nutrition is a vital aspect of helping these children discover, or recover, their full potential.

## Studies on the benefits of optimum nutrition

- Bernard Gesch, director of the charity Natural Justice, gave some of Britain's worst young offenders' supplements of vitamins, minerals and essential fats, or placebos, and demonstrated a dramatic 35 per cent decrease in aggressive acts only in those taking the supplements.[1] Another similar study is currently underway.

- Dr Alex Richardson of the University of Oxford conducted a randomised controlled trial with 117 children aged five to 12 years who had coordination problems. The children who received supplements of omega-3 and omega-6 essential fats showed significant improvements in reading, spelling and behaviour over three months compared to those who didn't receive the supplements.[2]

- Researchers from Örebro University in Sweden compared the school grades in ten core subjects with homocysteine levels (homocysteine is an indicator of B vitamin deficiency) in a group of 692 school children aged nine to 15. Higher homocysteine levels were strongly associated with lower grades.[3]

- Researchers at the Institute of Child Health in London placed 78 hyperactive children on a 'few foods' diet, which eliminated both chemical additives and common food allergens. The behaviour of 59 of the children, or 76 per cent, improved during this open trial. To check whether the foods would affect the children's behaviour if no one knew whether they were eating them or not, the researchers managed to disguise the foods and additives that provoked reactions in 19 of the children. When these children were given the disguised offending foods, their behaviour ratings and performance in psychological tests deteriorated.[4]

If simple changes in nutrition can have such profound effects on the young people in these studies, isn't it likely that optimum nutrition can help your child reach their full potential, whether they have behavioural problems, a condition such as autism or you feel they're doing 'all right'. As you follow the guidelines in this book, you'll notice gradual improvements in their ability to learn and behave. That's because you really can change how your child thinks, feels and behaves by changing what goes into their mouth – and we're going to show you how.

By doing so, you'll be in the vanguard of teachers, health professionals and other concerned parents who are leading a revolution in food awareness. Although governments are waking up to the implications of all the new research, they have not yet accepted across the board just how profoundly nutrition can influence learning and behaviour. In the UK, for example, over £240 million was spent last year on psychological interventions in school for children with learning or behavioural problems. How much was spent on the kind of highly effective nutritional intervention we describe in this book? Precisely nothing.

## How food builds the brain

One of the most limiting concepts in the human sciences is the idea that mind and body are separate. Try asking an anatomist, a psychologist and a biochemist where the mind begins and the body ends. It's a stupid question and yet that is exactly what modern science has done by separating psychology from medicine. Few psychologists know much about brain chemistry and the importance of nutrition, and few doctors know enough about the psychological or nutritional factors that affect a child's development.

However, it's not just the scientists who live by this false dichotomy. It's all of us. It's undoubtedly second nature to you to help your child grow physically strong and healthy, but when they're having difficulty concentrating, behaving badly or struggling to read, does the thought that they might be poorly nourished cross your mind? If it doesn't, it's vital to know that all these attributes and behaviours are governed by a network of interconnecting brain cells, each of which depends profoundly on what your child eats.

Many children struggle to keep up. They live with constant tiredness, difficulty in concentrating, erratic behaviour, anxiety, stress, depression and sleeping problems. Too many children suffer from mental health problems, ranging from attention deficit disorder to autism, hyperactivity and dyslexia; or they simply aren't achieving their full potential in school and at home, because the way they feel makes it difficult for them to focus and learn. In fact, all over the world there's been a massive rise in the incidence of mental health problems, especially among young people.[5]

By understanding how your child's brain works, you can eradicate these problems and smooth your child's path through their crucial developing years. It will become more than clear why giving a child certain nutrients every day, ideally from conception, can have a profound effect on how they think and feel, and thus how they behave in the here and now, and how they develop over time.

## Brains – what make us human

Our story starts not at birth, but at conception, and continues all the way through pregnancy. Studies of the time we spend in the womb show us that human growth and development – unlike that of, say, a rhinoceros – centre largely on the development of the brain. Brains, not brawn, are what make us human.

A rhino weights one tonne, but has a brain weighing 35g. A newborn baby weighs about 4kg, but has a brain weighing about 450g. A human baby's brain is more than 300 times larger, compared to its body size, than that of a rhinoceros, so size does matter – but that's not all. During development in the womb, half of all the nutrition the foetus receives from its mother is directly channelled into feeding brain growth.

This is quite a task. Although a mere 450g at birth, your child's brain consumes, and needs, a vast quantity of nutrients, including protein, carbohydrates, vitamins, minerals and essential fats. Fats are a big one here, as the brain is literally made out of it. In fact, if you drained all the water out of a brain, a whopping 60 per cent of what was left would be fat.

Four specific kinds of fat (known as AA, DHA, EPA and DGLA – more on these later) make up 20 per cent of the brain, so deficiencies of these at any time, but especially during foetal or early development, can have huge repercussions on intelligence and behaviour.

So vital are these fats to the growing foetus that it will literally rob its mother's brain to make its own. It's a case of 'Mummy, I shrunk your brain' and if a pregnant woman's diet is deficient in the essential fats, her brain will actually get smaller!

At every stage of brain development, achieving optimum nutrition is essential to guarantee that your child achieves their full potential. At birth, the level of essential fats in the umbilical cord of a newborn infant correlates with the speed of their thinking at age eight. By the age of eight, the blood level of homocysteine, which is the best indicator of a child's B vitamin status, will correlate with their school grades.[6] If a teenager's daily intake of zinc is just twice the level of the RDA, this can improve attention and concentration to an astonishing degree.[7] And at any age, a person's intake of anti-nutrients, such as sugar and damaged fats, has proven harmful effects on both learning and behaviour. If you find these facts hard to believe, you may not be aware of how flexible and open to change the human brain is. Let's look at it for a moment to fathom why this is.

## Joined-up thinking

As it grows, a foetus builds thousands of brain cells, called neurons, every minute. By the age of two, a child's brain has approximately 100 billion of them. That's a lot – approximately the same number of neurons as there are trees in the Amazon! Just like the interlocking branches of those billions of rainforest trees, the neurons

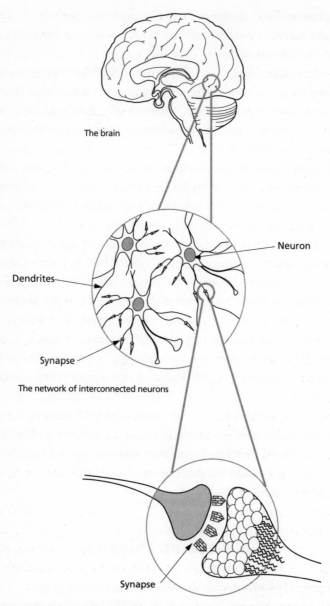

The brain

Dendrites

Neuron

Synapse

The network of interconnected neurons

Synapse

The synapse, where two cells meet

*The brain*

are connected up, so what we call the brain is essentially a network of these specialised nerve cells, all linked up to other neurons.

While the number of neurons doesn't increase in children beyond the age of two, the number of connections made between neurons does, very dramatically. When a baby is born, every neuron in the cerebral cortex – the 'grey matter' and outermost layer of the brain – can connect with about 2,500 other neurons. By the time that child is two or three years old, that number has swollen to 15,000. These connections are vital to memory, cognition and learning, because they're the conduits along which the electrical impulses of our thoughts travel, and children, those master learners, are hard-wiring these connections every minute.

When learning language, for instance, young children will keep repeating words to hard-wire the image they are seeing with the sound they are making, reinforced by your positive feedback. Every thought they think is represented by a 'ripple' of activity across the network of neurons. With repeated thoughts and actions, be it speech or movement, the neuronal pathways are reinforced. Meanwhile, redundant connections will get dismantled. Unlike other organs in the body, the brain is always restructuring itself.

Let's take a closer look at the connections between neurons. These are called dendrites and where one dendrite meets another there's a gap, like the 'spark' gap in a spark plug. This gap is called a synapse and it's across it that messages are sent from one neuron to another.

Messages are sent from a sending station and received in a receiving station, called a receptor. These sending and receiving stations are built out of essential fats, found in fish and seeds; phospholipids, present in eggs and organic meats; and amino acids, the raw material of protein.

The message itself, known as a neurotransmitter, is in most cases made out of amino acids. Different amino acids make different neurotransmitters. For example, the neurotransmitter serotonin, which keeps you happy, is made from the amino acid

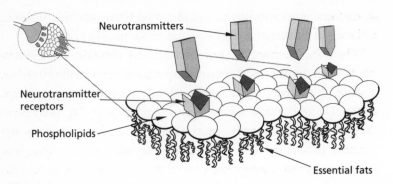

*Close-up on a receptor*

tryptophan. Adrenalin and dopamine, which keep you motivated, are made from phenylalanine.

Turning an amino acid into a neurotransmitter is no simple job. Enzymes in the brain that depend on vitamins, minerals and special amino acids accomplish this task. These vitamins and minerals also control the steady supply of fuel – blood sugar or glucose – that powers each neuron.

From all this, you can see how the food your children eat does more than build their bodies. It's building the very structure of their brains, from the neurons themselves to the messages that

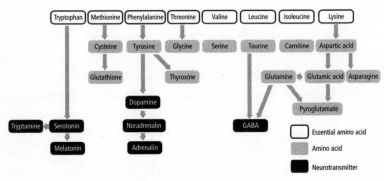

*Neurotransmitters are made from amino acids*

shoot from one to another, so food governs how your child thinks and feels to a massive degree.

The basic structure of your child's brain is laid down by genetics, but what you feed them, along with what they learn, helps develop that structure, and through that their intelligence, and ability to learn, adapt and have a happy, fulfilling life. While you can't change genes, you can change your child's nutrition and learning resources. That's why your biggest task as a parent is ensuring optimum nutrition, while stimulating your child's inbuilt capacity for learning.

Chapter 9

.

# Thinking faster, boosting IQ

First, we are all different due to our genes, and your child will inherit their own unique strengths and weaknesses. However, genes are less important than you might think and they are only part of the story when it comes to how your child develops. These bits of DNA are really just the instructions inside each cell to build proteins out of the amino acids that we eat. That means we inherit slightly different abilities to build certain proteins and that in turn changes not only how we look, but also how we think. That's because proteins make enzymes and enzymes make the neurotransmitters that are so key to how we think and feel. Since proteins, enzymes and neurotransmitters are all made from nutrients, it's no surprise to find that food directly affects the brain.

## The facets of intelligence

As we discussed in chapter 3, there are three kinds of intelligence: intellectual, emotional and physical. We are all well aware of intellectual intelligence which concerns your child's ability to learn, remember, solve problems, think laterally, concentrate and so on.

Emotional intelligence we can define as the ability to monitor one's own, and others' emotions, and react appropriately, channel our emotions to serve a goal, respond with empathy and maintain healthy relationships. Being sensitive to how another child feels and saying a kind word, not overreacting when things aren't going their own way or being able to say how they feel are all part of your child's emotional intelligence. Physical intelligence involves overall physical fitness, balance, agility and coordination, anticipation, reaction time, strength and flexibility. Not bumping into things and hurting yourself on a daily basis or being able to learn a physical skill are both examples of physical intelligence.

All these kinds of intelligence involve the brain, yet psychological and social theories of intelligence often seem to overlook this fundamental fact. Put simply, if your child's brain isn't working properly, they can't think or feel straight. Most of the problems we humans create in both our own and the larger world come about when we don't think clearly and then respond with inappropriate emotional reactions. To look at it another way, whatever your archetype of an 'enlightened' person might be – whether it's Buddha or Christ, Gandhi or the Dalai Lama, Einstein or Edison – the chances are that you define their enlightenment as an ability to think clearly and make measured responses.

However, are such qualities something we are born with or are they acquired? And do they depend in any way on nutrition? Even though there's obviously an inherited aspect to intelligence, we're going to show you how optimum nutrition promotes all-round intelligence by nourishing your child's brain.

It may surprise you to know that you can boost your child's intelligence quotient or IQ score at any age. Some people argue that your real 'intelligence' is innate, but the truth is that your ability to make intelligent decisions depends not only on this aspect of intelligence, but also on the clarity of your mind, how quickly you can think, your attention, how long you can concentrate and how good your memory is. All of these can be improved with optimum nutrition.

CASE HISTORY *Rachel, age 12*

At the age of four Rachel was diagnosed with global developmental delay and before she came to us at the Brain Bio Centre
her IQ was measured at 45 points. We assessed her nutrient
status and found that she was low in many key brain nutrients,
including zinc, magnesium and the B vitamins. Her diet simply did
not contain the nutrients that she needed. Improvements in her
diet, such as increasing the amount of freshly prepared food that
she ate and taking a high-dose multivitamin and mineral formula,
along with some fish oils, resulted in a 25-point increase in her
IQ after ten months.

The improvement seen in Rachel's case should not be surprising.
In part 1 we saw how the brain, composed of a highly complex network of neurons, is made from what we eat. Thinking is a pattern
of activity across this network. The messengers relaying the
thoughts are neurotransmitters, which again are made from, and
directly affected by, what we eat. When we learn, we actually
change the wiring of the brain. When we think, we change the
activity of neurotransmitters.

To a huge degree we and our children shape the way we think,
and this was the logic that made us investigate, in 1986, whether
giving a child an optimal intake of nutrients used by the brain and
nervous system would improve intellectual performance.

## Feeding the intellect

Way back in the early 1960s there was initial evidence of a link
between IQ and nutrition. Intellectual performance is generally
measured as IQ, with a score of 100 considered to be average.
About 5 per cent of children score above 125 and less than 10 per
cent score below 80, with such children considered to be in need
of special education help. A study in 1960 by Dr Albert Kubala and

his colleagues in the US showed that higher levels of vitamin C were associated with an increased IQ. Kubala divided 351 students into high and low vitamin C groups, depending on the levels of the vitamin in their blood. The students' IQ was then measured and found to average 113 and 109 respectively, with those with higher blood levels of vitamin C having IQs an average of 4.5 points higher.[1]

Then, in 1981, another researcher looked at the effect of multi-vitamins on children with learning disability. Having heard that some children with Down's syndrome had made big increases in IQ by taking multivitamins, Dr Ruth Harrell ran a trial that gave 22 learning disabled children high-strength multivitamin and mineral supplements or placebos.[2] After four months the IQs of the children taking the supplements had improved by between 5 and 10 points, while those on the placebo had shown no change. All the children were then put on the supplements and, after a further four months, the average IQ improvement was 10.2 points.

Again, in the early 1980s, we decided to test what would happen to the intelligence of children if they were given an optimal intake of vitamins and minerals. Gwillym Roberts, a schoolteacher and nutritional therapist from the Institute for Optimum Nutrition, and Professor David Benton, a psychologist from Swansea University, devised a test that put 60 children on to a special multivitamin and mineral supplement designed to ensure an optimal intake of key nutrients.[3] However, without their knowledge, half of these children took a placebo.

After eight months on the supplements, the non-verbal IQs in those taking the supplements had risen by over 10 points! No changes were seen in those on the placebos. This study, published in *The Lancet* in 1988, has since been proven many times in other studies. Most have used RDA levels of nutrients, which are much lower than those in our original study, but increases in IQ averaging 4.5 points have still been shown.

This now famous IQ study spawned more than a dozen similar studies to test the idea further. The next big one, conducted by professors Stephen Schoenthaler, John Yudkin, world-famous psychologist Hans Eysenck and Dr Linus Pauling, involved 615 children, who were given much lower RDA levels of nutrients. Once again, the results showed that the simple addition of a vitamin and mineral supplement could increase IQ scores by as much as 20 points, with an average increase of at least 4.5 points, this time over three months.[4]

The truth is that a 4.5 IQ point shift would get many thousands of educationally subnormal children reclassified and returned to mainstream schools. More comprehensive nutritional programmes have brought even children with IQs in the 40s back into the normal range, but your child doesn't have to be in this category to benefit, as children with high IQs have also shown improvement.

The results of our earlier trials have been replicated more than a dozen times and shown to work in ten out of 13 well-designed trials.[5] While most studies suggest that the children who are least well nourished benefit the most, two recent studies, in Australia and Indonesia, found that supplemental vitamins and minerals improved learning and memory even in well-nourished children.[6]

The consistent, positive benefit of giving your child supplements is also likely to last for life, according to a recent survey carried out by Aberdeen University's Department of Mental Health, which found that supplement use correlates with higher IQ scores later in life. This survey also emphasised the link between getting enough omega-3 fats and sharp intelligence.[7]

## How nutrients boost IQ

But how exactly do nutrients increase IQ scores? Wendy Snowden, a researcher from Reading University's psychology department, decided to investigate. Once again, children were given supplements or a placebo.[8] After ten weeks, the children taking supplements showed significant increases in non-verbal IQ scores, but not in verbal IQ scores. A close analysis of performance in the IQ tests showed the same proportion of errors, but the children were able to work faster and attempt more questions after the ten weeks of supplementation. For the verbal IQ test, all children completed all questions, so there was no room for improvement in work rate.

All this suggests that vitamin and mineral supplements effectively increase the speed of information processing in the brain – clearly a significant factor in IQ and, by implication, in intelligence. These amazing nutrients seem to help children think faster, and also concentrate for longer, which we'll explore in more detail in the next chapter.

## Go-faster food

Certain vitamins, minerals and fats seem particularly good at boosting brain speed. Let's look at them now.

### Brain-accelerating vitamins and minerals

When it comes to fast cognition, there is good reason to 'think zinc'. A recent trial involving 209 children aged ten to 11 in North Dakota showed remarkable results in how zinc supplements help speed up thinking.[9] The children were given a juice drink containing either 10mg of zinc, 20mg of zinc or none. The RDA for zinc for this age group is 10mg, so it's likely that these children would have been getting something like this level of the mineral.

At the beginning and end of the study, students had to perform a number of tests designed to measure mental skills, such as attention, memory, problem-solving and hand–eye coordination. Tasks included tapping a key on the keyboard as fast as possible, using a mouse to follow an object moving across the screen, searching a group of objects for two of a kind, learning and remembering lists of words or simple geometric patterns, and categorising objects.

Compared to the students who received no additional zinc, students given 20mg zinc each day decreased reaction time on a visual memory test by 12 per cent, versus 6 per cent; increased correct answers on a word recognition test by 9 per cent, versus 3 per cent;

and increased scores on a test requiring sustained attention and vigilance by 6 per cent, versus 1 per cent.

This illustrates why the RDA level of nutrients, which is the amount needed to prevent your child from developing a deficiency disease, such as scurvy from a lack of vitamin C, are hopelessly inadequate if you want to keep your child's brain optimally nourished. Other nutrients that boost IQ beyond RDA levels include vitamin B1, B6, B12, and folic acid. Studies with teenagers, for example, have found that 50mg of vitamin B1 a day improves speed of thinking[10] – yet the RDA is a mere 1.4mg!

So how much is enough? The RDA issue points to the need to know how much of the important vitamins and minerals your child requires to accelerate their thinking. Some die-hard dieticians still believe the mantra that your child 'can get all the nutrients they need from a well-balanced diet'. While we encourage you wholeheartedly to feed your child a well-balanced diet, as described in part 1, the evidence in dozens of studies reported in this book shows that achieving more than the basic RDA levels of nutrients will boost intelligence. In addition, our original study back in the mid-1980s, where children were given the highest levels of vitamins and minerals, produced the biggest increase in IQ scores.

The chart below shows the levels of vitamins and minerals that we recommend you give your child every day, assuming that you also ensure their diet is as good as it possibly can be, too.

## THE IDEAL DAILY SUPPLEMENT PROGRAMME: ESSENTIAL VITAMINS AND MINERALS

| Age | Less than 1 | 1–2 | 3–4 | 5–6 | 7–8 | 9–11 | 12–13 |
|---|---|---|---|---|---|---|---|
| **Vitamins** | | | | | | | |
| A (retinol) (mcg) | 500 | 650 | 800 | 1,000 | 1,500 | 2,000 | 2,500 |
| D (mcg) | 3 | 4 | 5 | 7 | 9 | 11 | 12 |
| E (mg) | 13 | 16 | 20 | 23 | 30 | 40 | 50 |
| C (mg) | 100 | 150 | 300 | 400 | 500 | 600 | 700 |

| Age | Less than 1 | 1–2 | 3–4 | 5–6 | 7–8 | 9–11 | 12–13 |
|---|---|---|---|---|---|---|---|
| B1 (thiamine) (mg) | 5 | 6 | 8 | 12 | 16 | 20 | 24 |
| B2 (riboflavin) (mg) | 5 | 6 | 8 | 12 | 16 | 20 | 24 |
| B3 (niacin) (mg) | 7 | 12 | 16 | 18 | 20 | 22 | 24 |
| B5 (pantothenic acid) (mg) | 10 | 15 | 20 | 25 | 30 | 35 | 40 |
| B6 (pyridoxine) (mg) | 5 | 7 | 10 | 12 | 16 | 20 | 25 |
| B12 (mcg) | 5 | 6.5 | 8 | 9 | 10 | 10 | 10 |
| Folic acid (mcg) | 100 | 120 | 140 | 160 | 180 | 200 | 220 |
| Biotin (mcg) | 30 | 45 | 60 | 70 | 80 | 90 | 100 |
| **Minerals** | | | | | | | |
| Calcium (mg) | 150 | 165 | 180 | 190 | 200 | 210 | 220 |
| Magnesium (mg) | 50 | 65 | 80 | 90 | 100 | 110 | 120 |
| Iron (mg) | 4 | 5.5 | 7 | 8 | 9 | 10 | 10 |
| Zinc (mg) | 4 | 5.5 | 7 | 8 | 9 | 10 | 10 |
| Manganese (mcg) | 300 | 350 | 400 | 500 | 700 | 1,000 | 1,000 |
| Iodine (mcg) | 40 | 50 | 60 | 70 | 80 | 90 | 100 |
| Chromium (mcg) | 15 | 19 | 23 | 25 | 27 | 30 | 30 |
| Selenium (mcg) | 10 | 18 | 20 | 24 | 26 | 28 | 30 |
| Copper (mcg) | 400 | 550 | 700 | 800 | 900 | 1,000 | 1,000 |

The easiest way to give your child all these vitamins and minerals is via a daily multi. The trouble with most multivitamin/mineral combinations is there aren't many good-tasting, chewable types that pack in these levels of nutrients. We've searched high and low, and list the ones worth buying (see page 295), including supplements that come in powder form or liquid drops that can be added to food and drinks. Of the chewable supplements, most involve taking, for example, one chewable tablet for every two years of life. So a six-year-old would take three a day.

## Essential fat – oiling the mental wheels

Back in the 1980s, the extent of supplementation for children was vitamins and minerals. Today we know that supplementing omega-3 fats is just as important. They not only improve your child's emotional intelligence and behaviour, they also keep those mental wheels well oiled, and running fast and smoothly.

The levels of omega-3 fats at birth, especially DHA, the 'brain-building' fat, predict intellectual development later in life,[11–12] and there is overwhelming evidence that supplementing DHA in infants improves the speed of their thinking and other measures of mental and physical performance at ages three,[13] four,[14] and seven[15]. So the effects of optimum nutrition during pregnancy and early infancy are long-lasting. Although not proven yet, it is highly likely that supplementation with fish oils rich in omega-3s throughout infancy and childhood will maximise a child's intellectual development.

Eating oily coldwater fish is an excellent way of getting more omega-3s into your child's diet and the chart below shows the amounts of DHA in each type. As we saw in chapter 3, however, be careful with tuna (go for the steaks, as the tinned variety has much less omega-3). It does tend to be high in mercury, so limit it to once every couple of weeks, and with salmon, stick with wild or organic farmed fish.

### BEST FISH FOR BRAIN FATS

Amount of DHA in 100g

| | |
|---|---|
| Mackerel | 1,400mg |
| Herring | 1,000mg |
| Sardines | 1,000mg |
| Tuna (steak, not tinned) | 900mg |
| Anchovy | 900mg |
| Salmon | 800mg |
| Trout | 500mg |

An ideal intake of DHA a day for your child is in the order of 300mg to 400mg a day, so if they're eating 100g of oily fish (preferably sardines, mackerel or herring) three times a week, they'll be doing very well. Alternatively, they can take a supplement of fish oils containing DHA. A good one can provide up to 200mg.

The best DHA source of all, at least for babies, is breast milk. It's naturally rich in DHA, particularly if the mother is eating fish or flaxseeds. Breast-fed babies not only have higher IQs ten years down the track[16] and better results in exams, they also have fewer mental health problems.[17]

In chapters 19 and 20 we'll show you some of the extraordinary results already achieved in children with ADHD and autism. You'll also learn how EPA, another kind of omega-3 fat abundant in fish oil, seems to help these children more than DHA. Hence we recommend that you supplement both DHA and EPA.

## THE IDEAL DAILY SUPPLEMENT PROGRAMME: OMEGA-3S

| Age | Less than 1 | 1–2 | 3–4 | 5–6 | 7–8 | 9–11 | 12–13 |
|---|---|---|---|---|---|---|---|
| *Essential fats* | | | | | | | |
| GLA (mg) | 50 | 75 | 95 | 110 | 135 | 135 | 135 |
| EPA (mg) | 100 | 175 | 250 | 300 | 350 | 350 | 350 |
| DHA (mg) | 100 | 140 | 175 | 200 | 225 | 225 | 225 |

Fish oils are the best way of supplementing omega-3s, but they're not to everyone's liking. Fortunately, nowadays there are many supplements, gels, oils and capsules cleverly flavoured to entice your child into developing the vital habit of supplementing fish oils every day.

Because oily fish can contain mercury, as we've pointed out, the fish oil supplements you give your child should be purified to be mercury-free. All those we list (see page 295) are not only free from mercury, but also come out best of those tested for the PCBs and other pollutants now sadly endemic in our seas.

## Summary

To maximise your child's IQ:

- Ensure an optimum intake of vitamins and minerals, both from diet and supplements, by giving your child a high-strength children's multivitamin and mineral supplement every day, not one based solely on the RDAs (see Products and Supplements Directory).

- Optimise your child's intake of essential fats, especially omega-3 fats, by giving them flaxseeds, oily fish and/or fish oil supplements every day.

# Chapter 10

# Developing concentration and a sharp memory

As a parent, you'll have seen at least one child who can't sit still, fidgets all the time and seems to lack a normal attention span. In fact, 'attention deficit' has become one of the most common problems afflicting today's children. Being able to stay focused on a task, project or piece of schoolwork is a key part of maximising a child's abilities. As we saw in the last chapter, achieving optimum nutrition through diet and supplements raises IQ partly because children concentrate better. Vitamins, however, aren't the key factor for concentration. It's sugar – or, more precisely, blood sugar balance.

## Blood sugar balance – the key to concentration

As we highlighted in chapter 2, keeping an even blood sugar level is critical to intelligence, because it's this, more than anything else, that affects your child's ability to concentrate over long periods of time. Why is that so? In a nutshell, it's all down to the brain's fuel, glucose – the sugar derived from the carbohydrates we eat. If, over time, your child eats too much of the wrong kind of carbohydrates, such as sweets and refined starchy foods, their blood and brain sugar levels start rollercoastering. When their blood sugar suddenly dips, their concentration can wander and any aggressive behaviour can get worse.[1-2]

This is why it's absolutely vital that your child eats a healthy breakfast and doesn't snack on sugary foods and drinks. A recent school survey found that almost two-thirds (65 per cent) of pupils eat sweets, chocolate bars or biscuits at least once a day; 64 per cent drink fizzy drinks or squashes that contain sugar; and 31 per cent eat chips or other fried potato snacks and crisps. All of these give your child a rush of sugar to their brain, followed abruptly by a sugar crash and poor concentration.

Aptos Middle School in San Francisco, California, took this message to heart and removed all sugared soft drinks from its vending machines. It also banned all refined carbohydrate snacks and foods, such as French fries, from the cafeteria. Since the nutrition changes were put into place, administrators and teachers report better student behaviour after lunch, fewer afternoon visits to the counselling office, less litter in the schoolyard and more students sitting down to eat. The school also reported higher scores on standardised tests. Its motto now? 'No empty calories!'

## The importance of eating breakfast

Many British schools have followed suit as a result of increased media attention and new guidelines from the UK's School Food Trust. Others have set up 'breakfast clubs' to encourage children who don't eat breakfast to get into the habit of having it. If that sounds peculiar to you, because your kids always leave the house set up by a plate of eggs or a bowl of porridge, you should know that a third of children in Britain don't have a proper breakfast, but, according to a number of studies,[3] those who do have much better concentration and attention spans.

Breakfast should become a golden rule in any household, but

what reaches the table needs some thought. For instance, school breakfast clubs are a great idea, but some reportedly serve sugary cereals or golden syrup on white toast, so if your child attends one it's vital to check and see what's on the menu.

The best breakfast is a low-GL one. As we saw in chapter 2, low-GL carbohydrates are the kind that keep your child's blood sugar even. Cereal is an easy and deservedly popular breakfast choice, but one with a number of pitfalls, because few commercial cereals are low-GL. Let's look at the options in the chart below.

## GLYCAEMIC LOAD OF BREAKFAST CEREALS

| Food | Serving size in g | Looks like | GL per serving |
|------|------------------|------------|----------------|
| Low-carb muesli (see *The Low-GL Diet Cookbook*) | 60 | Large bowl | 4 |
| Porridge made from rolled oats | 30 | Large bowl | 2 |
| GoodCarb Original Granola | 50 | Medium bowl | 5 |
| Get Up & Go (made with water) | 30 | ½ pint drink | 3 |
| Get Up & Go with strawberries and ½ pint of milk | 30 | ½ pint drink | 8.5 |
| All-Bran™ | 30 | 1 small serving | 6 |
| Muesli, gluten-free | 30 | 1 medium serving | 7 |
| Muesli (Alpen) | 30 | 1 serving | 10 |
| Muesli, natural | 30 | 1 serving | 10 |
| Raisin Bran™ (Kellogg's) | 30 | 1 medium serving | 12 |
| Weetabix™ | 25 | 2 biscuits | 11 |
| Bran Flakes™ | 30 | 1 medium serving | 13 |
| Sultana Bran™ (Kellogg's) | 30 | 1 medium serving | 14 |
| Special K™ (Kellogg's) | 30 | 1 medium serving | 14 |
| Shredded Wheat™ | 40 | 2 biscuits | 20 |
| Cheerios™ | 30 | 1 medium serving | 15 |
| Frosties™ (Kellogg's) | 30 | 1 medium serving | 15 |
| Grapenuts™ | 30 | 1 medium serving | 15 |
| Golden Wheats™ (Kellogg's) | 30 | 1 medium serving | 16 |
| Puffed Wheat | 30 | 1 medium serving | 16 |

continues →

| Food | Serving size in g | Looks like | GL per serving |
|------|-------------------|------------|----------------|
| Honey Smacks™ (Kellogg's) | 30 | 1 medium serving | 16 |
| Cornflakes, Crunchy Nut™ (Kellogg's) | 30 | 1 medium serving | 17 |
| Coco Pops™ | 30 | 1 medium serving | 20 |
| Rice Krispies™ (Kellogg's) | 30 | 1 medium serving | 21 |
| Cornflakes™ (Kellogg's) | 30 | 1 medium serving | 21 |

It depends on your child's age, size and activity levels, but the general goal is for breakfast to have a GL of around ten, including added fruit, so ideally the cereal part should have a GL of around five. As you can see, that rules out almost every branded cereal. This is especially true when you look at the quantity of cereal the recommended serving size provides, which in many cases is ludicrously small.

The Consumers' Association checked out 28 branded cereals and found that nine contained 40 per cent or more sugar! The worst options included Quaker Sugar Puffs™, which contained 49g per 100g, and Frosties™. In fact, a bowl of Frosties™ contained the equivalent of four heaped teaspoons of sugar. Don't forget – when you're checking the label, there are many different names for added sugar to look out for, including honey, malt, fructose, dextrose, glucose and inverted glucose syrup. From the point of view of sugar content, the best packaged cereal was Weetabix ReadyBrek™.

The best breakfast cereal option by far is porridge oat flakes, which can be eaten hot and cooked or cold and raw, sweetened with fresh fruit. GoodCarb Original Granola is also excellent, as is Low GL Get Up and Go, a breakfast shake powder that you blend with milk and berries. Alternatively, you could make your own low-GL muesli with oats, seeds, nuts and oat bran, and sweeten your child's daily portion with fresh fruit. However, you don't have to give your child cereal. Ring the changes with high-protein, low-GL and thoroughly delectable options such as eggs or kippers, both of which can be served with wholegrain toast (see chapter 22 for more on breakfasts).

## Grazing the low-GL way

Eating low-GL, slow-releasing carbohydrates and grazing, not gorging, is the best way to avoid blood sugar dips, so it's good to encourage healthy snacking from the start by having a bountiful bowl of fruit available at all times. The best fruits are apples, pears, peaches and berries, from strawberries to blueberries. Provided your child is not too young to be nibbling on nuts or seeds, a handful of pumpkin seeds, sunflower seeds or almonds is also a great snack. As far as school is concerned, you can always send your child to school armed with an apple, and a tub of nuts and seeds.

Other good snacks are oat cakes. Choose rough oat cakes that are sugar-free, because these have the lowest GL score. You can also buy oat biscuits which, although they do contain sugar, have a fraction of that found in other biscuits; so they're good as a treat. It's also an excellent idea to have a non-sugary spread, such as peanut (or any other nut) butter, in your store cupboard. A teaspoon spread on an oat cake makes for a delicious, sustaining and healthy snack.

## Farewell to the fizz

The worst offenders, as far as sugar is concerned, are sweet, fizzy drinks. A 2 litre bottle of cola contains more than 40 teaspoons of sugar! Most of this category of drinks are best avoided. The best drink to encourage is water: if a child is brought up drinking water when thirsty, that is what they'll drink. Of all the fruit juices, apple, pear and orange are best, but, as we've already said, make sure you pick 100 per cent fresh fruit juices, dilute them at least half and half with water, and don't make them a staple. Avoid products called 'fruit juice drinks' as these inevitably contain added sugar.

## Natural memory boosters

Concentration is one thing, but once your child has finished a task, what about their recall of it? Memory is vital in school and beyond. Let's look at which nutrients are key in this context.

### Phosphatidyl choline

The main brain chemical involved in memory is called acetyl-choline and to make it your child needs the phospholipid called phosphatidyl choline (PC). As we saw in chapter 3, the richest dietary sources of PC are egg yolks and fish, especially sardines. A child needs about 500mg to 1,000mg of PC a day to maximise mental function. Most lecithin supplements contain about 20 per cent PC, so your child ideally needs 2.5g to 5g of lecithin a day. You can also buy high-PC lecithin, which is twice as rich in PC, so your child would only need 1g to 2.5g, or a level teaspoon, of this a day.

However, PC isn't the only substance you need to make more acetylcholine. Vitamin B5 (pantothenic acid) is also essential for the formation of acetylcholine in the body, as are vitamins B1[4–5], B12 and also vitamin C, so memories are made of a good multivitamin, too.

Research reveals that taking PC during pregnancy can result in offspring with 'superbrains',[6] but supplementing PC later on helps children and adults alike. Dr Ladd and colleagues at the West Valley College in Saratoga, California, gave 80 students a single 25g dose of PC and found a significant improvement in memory 90 minutes later, probably due to the improved responses of slow learners.[7] If you combine PC with other 'smart' nutrients such as pyroglutamate (see page 124), you can achieve the same memory-boosting effect at lower amounts.

### Phosphatidyl serine

Phosphatidyl serine (PS) is another phospholipid essential to memory and, like PC, it's found in eggs and organic meats. Along with essential fats and protein, PS is one of the main materials used in the 'docking ports' on neurons – the receptor sites where neurotransmitters latch on to deliver their messages. As such, PS is very important to the smooth working of your child's brain.

## DMAE

DMAE is another substance that's needed to make acetylcholine and one of its features is that it crosses very easily from the blood into the brain cells, accelerating the brain's production of acetylcholine. DMAE reduces anxiety, stops the mind racing, improves concentration, promotes learning and acts as a mild brain stimulant, and sardines, once again, are a rich source of it.

The ideal dose of DMAE for memory enhancement is 100mg for children under seven and up to 500mg for teenagers, taken in the morning or at midday, but not last thing at night. Too much DMAE can overstimulate and it's therefore not recommended for people diagnosed with schizophrenia, mania or epilepsy. Don't expect its effect to be immediate, though. DMAE can take two to three weeks to work, but the results are worth waiting for.

## Glutamine and pyroglutamate – amazing brain fuel

While acetylcholine is the major player as far as memory is concerned, many neurotransmitters are also involved. Some stimulate mental processes, while others prevent information overload, and, unsurprisingly, a good balance works best. For example, the neurotransmitter GABA, which is made from the amino acid glutamine, helps forge links between memories and calms down an overexcited nervous system. However, a slight variation in this key memory molecule, called glutamate, can literally overexcite neurons to death if there is too much of it 'free' or unbound in the bloodstream. Indeed, this is how MSG or monosodium glutamate turns up your tastebuds.

Another form of this amino acid, pyroglutamate, greatly enhances learning. Pyroglutamate is found in many foods, including fish, dairy products, fruits and vegetables. What pyrogluamate does is increase acetylcholine production, boost the number of receptors for acetylcholine and improve communication between the left and right hemispheres of the brain. In other words, it enhances the brain's ability to 'talk and listen', and improves cooperation between the two hemispheres. As a result, learning, memory, concentration and the speed of reflexes will all benefit.

Glutamine is the most abundant amino acid in the cerebrospinal fluid surrounding the brain. It can be used directly as fuel for the brain and has been shown to enhance mood and mental performance, and decrease addictive tendencies.[8] In studies designed to test whether glutamine proved safe in large doses, researchers from Boston Women's Hospital in Massachusetts gave healthy volunteers between 40g and 60g a day. Not only was it shown to be safe, but one of the side-effects was an enhanced ability to solve problems on continuous performance tests. This study was only five days long, but it demonstrated that glutamine has an immediate effect and may have a greater effect over time.[9]

Glutamine is an important nutrient for the brain and there is good logic to adding 500mg to 1,000mg, depending on age, to your child's daily supplement programme, especially if they are having learning problems. However, some children, particularly those on the autistic spectrum have a problem processing glutamine. In this case, glutamine can cause over stimulation and excess production of ammonia. As a precaution, do not give glutamine to an autistic child unless under the direct supervision of a qualified nutritional therapist. Glutamine can be bought in powder form; some supplements contain either glutamine or pyroglutamate. As with all the other brain nutrients we've discussed in this chapter – PC, PS and DMAE – it's best taken in the morning as it has a stimulating effect on your child's mental function.

## Summary

To improve your child's concentration and memory:

- Always give your child a healthy, low-GL breakfast.

- Encourage snacking on fruit, nuts, seeds, oat cakes or, in moderation, oat biscuits.

- Avoid sugary drinks, choosing water and half-and-half diluted juices instead.

- Add a level teaspoon of lecithin, high in phosphatidyl choline, or a dessertspoon of regular lecithin, to your child's cereal each morning.

- Alternatively, consider giving your child a supplement that contains a combination of the brain food nutrients listed above – phosphatidyl choline, phosphatidyl serine, DMAE and pyroglutamate.

# Chapter 11

·

# Revving up reading and writing

At the age of five, some kids are just learning their letters and others are reading Hans Christian Andersen. There are huge differences, too, in their progress with pencil and paper. All this is perfectly natural. When it comes to reading and writing, children develop at their own pace. They all take a different length of time and have a different natural aptitude for these vital skills. There can be a gender difference, too, as boys often develop later in this regard. However, having said this, if your child struggles with reading or writing and is behind at school, you may be able to help them by improving their nutrition.

## CASE HISTORY *Reece, age 7*

Reece couldn't sit still for long, had decided he didn't like reading and was behind at school. His mother had taken him to a psychologist, but that hadn't helped. When we met Reece and his mother we encouraged them to carry out a one-week 'experiment' in which Reece was to be given ground seeds on his cereal, more fish, less meat, no sugar or foods with chemical additives, and a special drink called Optio, which is the equivalent of a multivitamin and mineral in a fruit juice.

One week later, not only did Reece write one and a half pages in the same amount of time as he had previously written four lines, but his handwriting also improved dramatically. His mother, who was sceptical about the trial, said, 'I thought that nothing could calm this child down. He was very fidgety, he was hard to get into bed, hyperactive, constantly on the go and with occasional tantrums. Now he's a completely different child. He's a lot calmer and he wants to do more at school. In two weeks his reading has gone up a level. He doesn't get so overexcited and he's much nicer to be with. We're definitely going to stick with the diet.'

At the end of the first month, Reece's reading level had gone up a year. He now loves reading and his writing is improving in leaps and bounds.

Problems with reading and writing are often due to perceptual difficulties, so one of the first things to rule out is short- or long-sightedness. Often children who struggle to read and write simply have poor eyesight. Improving their eyesight with natural vision methods, such as the Bates Method (see page 295), can bring considerable improvement. Alternatively, get them tested for glasses. However, just as often, the problem lies not in the ability of the eyes to focus, but in the ability of the brain to process the information correctly.

An extreme example of this is dyslexia. If you are concerned that your child might have dyslexia and know that there's a history of literacy difficulties in your family, complete the following questionnaire.

## DYSLEXIA CHECK

Check whether your child has symptoms of dyslexia by answering the questions below. To answer some of these questions you may need to see your child in the classroom and/or consult their teacher.

Is your child...

- [ ] a relatively late speaker compared to other children of their age?

- [ ] good at things with a strong visual element, but inexplicably poor in other set tasks?

- [ ] showing evidence of laterality confusion – do they do some things, such as write or kick a ball, with the left and some things with the right side?

- [ ] unable to follow a number of instructions in a sequence, such as 'Go to the bedroom, get my slippers, then bring them to me'?

- [ ] writing reversed letters or numbers?

- [ ] having particular difficulty with literacy or one area of literacy, such as spelling or reading?

- [ ] noticeably inconsistent when reading – recognising words, then being unable to read the same word later in the page, book or day?

- [ ] not spotting words spelt correctly when offered a range of spellings for the same word?

- [ ] often spelling the same word in different ways on the same page and, if asked the difference between the various spellings, unable to identify them?

- [ ] when engaged in literacy tasks, taking a noticeably different time to do them than other tasks, such as drawing or practical activities?

☐ able to give an answer verbally or read out a story, but producing little when asked to write it?

☐ described by others as clumsy?

☐ unable to add a rhyming or alliterative word to a sequence of rhyming or alliterative words?

☐ on a much easier reading book than most of their close friends?

☐ in a much lower spelling group than most of their close friends?

☐ showing a marked difference compared to the rest of their class during note-taking or a copying activities?

☐ showing a noticeable difference in work output if given help with planning their work?

☐ producing more work, and generally seeming much happier at school, if taught strategies to develop sequencing skills?

☐ beginning to resist writing because they are bad at it?

☐ looking up at the board during a copying activity much more often than the children around them?

☐ responding to a handwriting development programme?

☐ over time, losing confidence when in educational settings?

☐ complaining that 'the words move around on the page' when he or she is trying to read?

*If you answer 'yes' to a lot of these questions, you should see an educational psychologist, who can determine whether your child has dyslexia.*

## Dyslexia and dyspraxia

Children with dyslexia experience specific problems in learning to read and write, sometimes because of subtle variations in visual perception. Difficulties in arithmetic and reading musical notation are also common, as are poor working memory, problems with deciphering the sounds of words and a faulty sense of direction.

Around 5 per cent of the population is severely dyslexic, although many more are affected by milder forms of the condition. If you've completed the check above and suspect your child might be dyslexic, you should speak to your child's teacher or head teacher. Many schools have special needs teachers who can assess your child thoroughly. If your child's school doesn't do this, contact the Dyslexia Action (see Resources). It can put you in touch with an educational psychologist who can carry out this assessment.

Getting your child assessed is useful on a number of counts. It helps them become aware that they have a difficulty, allows them to work with a special needs teacher to minimise the problem, and gives them special privileges, such as more time for exams and the use of computers at school.

Recent research suggests that pure dyslexia – that is, substantially delayed reading and writing in otherwise bright children – may have to do with a subtle brain difference in how these children perceive the 'small sounds', or phonetical building blocks, of words. This makes it harder for them to both read and understand word meanings, as they simply don't have a good grip on the basics. Special teaching techniques to compensate for this can dramatically improve your child's reading and writing skills.

Less well known, but equally prevalent, dyspraxia involves poor coordination and difficulties in carrying out complex sequenced actions. Children with the condition find it hard to catch a ball, tie shoelaces or do up buttons, but, more seriously, their handwriting can be extremely difficult to read, and they can experience real difficulties with organisation, attention and concentration. On top of assessments and tailored teaching, children with dyslexia and dyspraxia can benefit massively from the right nutrition.

## Eat for vision and coordination

Whether your child has dyslexia, dyspraxia or is just struggling with their 'three Rs', you'll want to maximise nutrients that will help their brain and eyes, and when it comes to that, oily fish and carrots are the dynamic duo.

### Essential fats – seeing is believing

We discussed the importance of essential fats for proper brain function in chapter 3 and a high concentration of essential fats is also needed by the eyes, so that they can manage the very rapid movements associated with vision. Children with dyslexia, dyspraxia and learning difficulties are very often deficient in these essential fats and/or the nutrients needed to properly utilise them, and the benefits of increasing the intake of these fats have been clearly documented in many studies.[1–2]

A study of 97 dyslexic children by Dr Alex Richardson at Hammersmith Hospital in London revealed that essential fat deficiency clearly contributes to the severity of dyslexic problems. Those children with the worst essential fat deficiencies showed significantly poorer reading and lower general ability than the non-deficient children.[3]

So how do you know if your child is deficient in essential fats? You could start with our Fat check (see chapter 3), but a key indicator is dry skin or eczema. In fact, in a study of 60 children at the Royal London Hospital, Dr Christine Absolon and her colleagues found twice the rate of 'psychological disturbance' in children with eczema, compared to those without.[4]

If your child has some of the outward symptoms of essential fat deficiency – rough dry patches on the skin, cracked lips, dull or dry hair, soft or brittle nails and excessive thirst – it's fair to say that this could be contributing to any concentration or visual problems, mood swings, disturbed sleep patterns and in some cases behavioural problems they may have. This is because dyslexia, dyspraxia, learning difficulties and ADHD all involve poor nerve cell communications in the brain and essential fats are crucial in keeping neurons talking to each other.[5]

To test the value of supplementing essential fats in dyspraxia, Dr Jacqueline Stordy of the University of Surrey in the UK gave essential fat supplements containing DHA, EPA, AA and DGLA to 15 children whose performance on standardised measures of motor and coordination skills placed them in the bottom 1 per cent of the population. After 12 weeks of supplementation, they all showed significant improvements in manual dexterity, ball skills, balance and parental ratings of their dyspraxic symptoms.[6] Stordy also assessed the benefit of essential fat supplementation in dyslexia and found that, after just four weeks of supplementation with EPA and DHA, their night vision and dark adaptation (which are usually very poor in dyslexics) had completely normalised.[7] Of course, it's just as vital for kids to avoid fried and hydrogenated fats as it is to top up their essential fats.

## The As have it

We've seen that the eyes need plenty of omega-3 fats, but they also require vitamin A. In fact, vitamin A is so vital to vision that its name, retinol, is a direct reference to its role in keeping the retina working properly. (Retinol is the animal form of vitamin A, found in meat, fish and eggs; beta-carotene, the vegetable form, is converted into retinol in the liver.) Some fish oil supplements, notably cod liver oil, contain both vitamin A as retinol and omega-3 fats, so if you suspect your child's problems with reading or writing are down to vision problems, you could try giving them this kind of supplement for a month.

With vitamin A, however, it's vital to know safe limits, as it's one of the few vitamins that can be stored in the body and in very large amounts can cause problems. For instance, during pregnancy a woman taking more than 5,000mcg a day may increase the risk of birth defects in her child. For your child, the ideal amount is much less than this – between 500mcg and 2,000mcg, depending on your child's age (see chapter 9). The table below shows much your child would need to eat to achieve 500mcg.

**VITAMIN A IN FOODS**

| Type of food | Amount giving 500mcg of vitamin A (as retinol) |
| --- | --- |
| Liver | 4g |
| Whole milk | 160g |
| Cheddar cheese | 160g |
| Parmesan cheese | 240g |
| Cream cheese | 110g |
| Egg | 6 eggs |
| Butter | 11 tablespoons |
| Mackerel | 900g |
| Kidney | 130g |
| Chicken | 1.6kg |

Of course, no one is going to eat that much chicken, mackerel, butter or egg at one sitting, but it's important to know how much vitamin A your child's food contains, so you can balance that out with all other sources of vitamin A and ensure that the total amount of vitamin A doesn't exceed double the optimum daily supplemental for your child's age. Most multivitamins will contain some retinol, usually in the region of 500mcg. Cod liver oil capsules vary considerably, though, so do check the label – most will provide between 500 and 1,000mcg per capsule.

## Pesticides – bad news for the eyes

When the eye is processing visual information, it turns vitamin A into rhodopsin, a light-sensitive pigment. Light reaching the rhodopsin reacts with it, after which the pigment undergoes a cycle of changes that, effectively, recycles it back into rhodopsin. This cycle is particularly important for black and white vision, which is for the most part what we use at night, which is why your grandmother told you carrots would help you see in the dark. Organophosphate pesticides and herbicides, now being phased out in most developed countries, but still used widely in developing countries, block this conversion. While this is unlikely to be a significant factor in your child's visual ability, it does highlight why it is so important to keep our children free from such chemicals, so keep choosing organic food whenever you can (see chapter 6).

Sugar also worsens eye movement in dyslexics, too. A study of people with dyslexia found that a poor diet, high in sugar, caused more erratic eye movements, while a good diet, without sugar, caused 'normal' eye movements.[8]

## Summary

To support your child's reading and writing:

- Ensure they're getting an optimal intake of nutrients from their diet as well as a good-quality multivitamin/mineral supplement with enough zinc.

- Minimise your child's intake of sugar.

- Ensure an optimal intake of essential fats from seeds, their cold-pressed oils and oily fish, plus sufficient antioxidants, especially vitamin E, to protect them from free-radical damage.

- Ensure an optimum intake of vitamin A from food, supplements and fish oil capsules.

- Minimise your child's intake of fried food, processed food, and saturated fat from meat and dairy.

- Keep your child 'chemical-free' by choosing organic food whenever possible.

# PART 3

·

# SOLVING PROBLEMS

In this part of the book we'll show you how to address the most common health problems experienced by children today.

# Chapter 12

·

# Obesity and being overweight

Obesity is a modern problem – statistics for it did not even exist 50 years ago. Figures from the World Health Organization show that at least 20 million children under the age of five are overweight globally. The figures for the UK are no less alarming. According to the NHS, the number of obese children has tripled over the last 20 years. At least 10 per cent of six-year-olds and 17 per cent of 15-year-olds are now clinically obese. Childhood obesity is not 'puppy fat'. In previous generations, a chubby child could be expected to slim naturally in adolescence, but for the current generation of children this no longer holds. Childhood obesity is a strong indicator of adult obesity and is likely to lead to serious health risks in later life.

If your child is overweight, they are more likely to experience low self-esteem, have an unhealthy relationship with food, and be at risk of serious diseases such as type II diabetes and fatty liver disease. As they get older, they are at a much higher risk of heart disease, cancer, arthritis, diabetes and metabolic syndrome (this has four major components – obesity, high blood pressure, high cholesterol and fats in the blood, and diabetes). As they get older, of course, they will also find it more difficult to lose weight.

## Is your child overweight?

The standard measure of overweight or obesity in adults is the body mass index (BMI), a calculation of weight in kilograms per square metre of height. However, adult BMI isn't appropriate for children, since BMI changes markedly as a child ages. A certain BMI at one age may be the norm, but for another age the same BMI may be unusually high or low. So how do you know if your child is overweight or obese? For children, BMI is converted into centiles, using reference data based on sex and age. These centiles can then be used to categorise BMI. For example, a child in the 95th centile or above is classed as obese. If you are concerned about your child's weight, you should speak to your health visitor or GP who can tell you where your child sits on the scale and what it means.

## What causes overweight and obesity in children?

Conventional wisdom tells us that children are overweight because they eat too much and don't do enough exercise, but this is a simplistic assessment of the problem. For some children, genetics may play a part. Often, though, if being overweight tends to run in the family it is just as likely that it's due to the similar dietary and lifestyle habits of family members. There's some evidence that obesity may start in the womb. Higher birth weight babies born to women who are obese during pregnancy are more likely to develop metabolic syndrome[1], and children who are breast-fed more than bottle-fed or breast-fed for a longer period are less likely to become overweight or obese.[2] All these factors may contribute towards excess weight gain in a child, but in truth it comes down to what a child eats rather than how much.

As with adults, evidence is gathering that the main dietary component that contributes to overweight and obesity is sugar rather than fat. As we saw in chapter 2, fast releasing high-GL carbohydrates – in other words refined starchy foods and sugar – cause dramatic rises in blood sugar level and this excess sugar is then stored as fat.

## Fighting the flab

Children who eat a naturally healthy diet that is rich in nutrients and delivers a low GL, and who lead a moderately active life, will not have issues with their weight. It's as simple as that. If your child is overweight or obese, focus on eating healthily, for all the compelling reasons that we've outlined in part 1 of this book. Low-fat diets and calorie-counting are unsuitable for children and lead to a poor relationship with food. In addition, if you struggle with your own weight, you'll need to set the right example for your child, so look at your own attitude to food, too (see part 4 for more on this).

There's also no doubt that declining levels of activity are contributing to the obesity epidemic in both adults and children. Children are much less likely to walk or cycle to school than their parents, time dedicated to physical activity in school is in decline and many children return from a day of sitting at school to spending the evening doing homework, watching television, playing computer games and eating. Different types of exercise will appeal to different children, so work together with your child to find something they will enjoy. Some children will enjoy a team sport or a dance class, while others might be happiest taking the dog for a daily brisk walk. Could your children join a 'walking bus' to get to school? Setting the right example is essential here as well, and remember that exercise not only improves health, it lifts mood too, so it could be the ideal thing for your moody teenager.

## A good night's sleep to fight the flab

Finally – and this is particularly interesting – according to a US study a good night's sleep may reduce your child's risk of becoming obese.[3] Dr Julia Lumeng from Michigan University analysed the sleep patterns of 785 children from ten US cities and took measures of their weight and height. Of the children who slept ten to 12 hours each night at age eight, around 12 per cent were obese by age 11. Twice as many children who slept less than nine hours were obese by the same age. Dr Lumeng speculates that it could be because tired children are less likely to go out and play. However, the study does tally with several others, some of which have found that hormonal changes brought on by a lack of sleep can lead to an increased appetite, particularly for sweet and starchy foods (see chapter 17 for more on sleep).

## Summary

To tackle your child's weight problems:

- Ensure they're eating an optimum nutrition diet (see part 4 for more on this).

- Blood sugar balance is especially important to achieve and maintain a healthy weight.

- Don't follow overly restrictive diets such as low-fat, or calorie-counting regimes – focus on eating for health as a family.

- Ensure your child is active every day, whether that be playing sport or walking the dog.

# Chapter 13

# Protecting your child from food allergies

As many as one in five adults and children,[1-2] and probably one in three with behavioural problems, are sensitive or have allergic reactions to common foods, such as milk, wheat, yeast and eggs. Yet the knowledge that allergy to foods and chemicals can adversely affect a child's health has been ignored for a very long time.

Back in the 1980s, researchers found that allergies can affect any system of the body and be behind a diverse range of symptoms, from fatigue, eczema, asthma, aching joints, constipation, diarrhoea, tummy aches and frequent ear infections, to slowed thought processes, irritability, agitation, aggressive behaviour, nervousness, anxiety, depression, ADHD, autism, hyperactivity and learning disabilities.[3-4]

## CASE HISTORY *Veronica, age five*

Veronica had been diagnosed with mild autism and also suffered her entire life from chronic constipation and regular tummy aches. When her parents brought her to us at the Brain Bio Centre, we arranged an IgG (see page 143) food allergy test that revealed an allergy to gluten. When this was removed from her diet, her parents were pleased to report a major improvement in her sociability and much improved digestion, with regular bowel movements and no tummy aches.

The most convincing evidence for the wide-ranging effects of food allergies comes from a well-conducted trial by Dr Joseph Egger and his team, who studied 76 hyperactive children to find out whether diet could contribute to behavioural disorders. The results showed that 79 per cent of the children tested reacted adversely to artificial food colourings and preservatives, primarily tartrazine and benzoic acid, which produced a marked deterioration in their behaviour.

However, Egger found that no child reacted to these alone. In fact, among the children tested, 48 different foods were found to produce symptoms. For example, 64 per cent reacted to cow's milk, 59 per cent to chocolate, 49 per cent to wheat, 45 per cent to oranges, 39 per cent to eggs, 32 per cent to peanuts and 16 per cent to sugar. Interestingly, it was not only the children's behaviour that improved after their diets were modified. Most of the associated symptoms also lessened considerably, including headaches, fits, abdominal discomfort, chronic rhinitis, aches in limbs, skin rashes and mouth ulcers.[5] Other studies have reported very similar results.[6]

These studies show how problems created by allergies often produce a multitude of physical and mental symptoms, and affect many systems within the body. Furthermore, allergies, and the symptoms they create, are very specific to the individual.

## Allergy, intolerance or sensitivity?

These days, people use the terms food allergies, food intolerances and food sensitivities almost interchangeably. So what is the difference? The classic definition of an allergy is simply an exaggerated physical reaction to a substance where the immune system is clearly involved. The immune system, which is the body's defence system, has the ability to produce 'markers' for substances it doesn't like, the classic example being an antibody called IgE (immunoglobulin type E). When food meets its IgE marker, it triggers the release of chemicals. These include histamine, which causes the classic symptoms of allergy – skin rashes, hay-fever, rhinitis, sinusitis, asthma, eczema and anaphylaxis (a reaction whereby the throat and mouth swell, accompanied by a severe asthma attack and sometimes a rash, a rapid drop in blood pressure, an irregular heartbeat and loss of consciousness). All of these 'IgE-mediated' reactions are immediate and severe, and may be life-threatening and lifelong. If your child has this type of allergy, you probably already know about it and are keeping your child well away from the offending food.

However, the most common type of food allergy involves a different marker – IgG. Often called 'delayed-onset', because the reactions may take anywhere from an hour to three days to show themselves, the symptoms of IgG allergies are usually  relatively undramatic, but they do affect many systems of the body. Add to this the fact that IgG reactions are often to a number of common foods and your child may well end up eating foods they're allergic to on a regular basis, without you knowing it.

Food intolerances and sensitivities are reactions to food where there is no measurable immune response. Examples of these include lactose intolerance, where a child lacks the enzyme to digest milk sugar (lactose) and can develop diarrhoea and abdominal discomfort when they drink milk; or sensitivity to the flavour enhancer MSG, which makes some kids hyperactive, although the mechanism behind the reaction is not understood.

## The top ten allergens

Any food can cause an allergic reaction, but the most common include wheat and other gluten grains, milk and milk products, eggs, foods containing yeast, shellfish, nuts, peanuts, garlic and soya. Most food allergies are a reaction to the protein in a particular food, particularly the foods that are eaten most frequently.

Wheat is probably top of this list, because it contains a substance called gliadin, which irritates the gut wall. Gliadin is a type of gluten, a sticky protein that allows pockets of air to form when combined with yeast, hence it allows bread dough to rise. Eating a lot of wheat products isn't good for anyone and especially not for your child if they have an allergy to them. The connections between wheat allergy, autism and ADHD are well established (see chapters 19 and 20 for more on this).

Rye, barley and oats contain much less gluten, as well as different types of it, so if your child is allergic to wheat, they may be able to tolerate rye, barley and oats. Some children who are allergic to wheat, rye and barley can only tolerate oats, which contains no gliadin.

Dairy products, including cheese and yoghurt, cause allergic reactions in many children. Some children seem to be able to tolerate goat's or sheep's milk, but not cow's milk. However, this could in part be because if they cut out cow's milk they simply consume less dairy overall, as goat's and sheep's milk and cheese tend to come in smaller cartons and blocks and are not so easily obtainable. Allergic reactions often include a blocked nose, frequent colds, bloating and indigestion, 'thick' head, fatigue, earaches and headaches.

## Getting to grips with allergies

Let's take a look at the options for investigating whether food allergies are causing problems for your child.

### Allergy tests

If your child has a history of infantile colic, eczema, asthma, ear or chest infections, hay-fever, seasonal allergies, digestive problems (including bloating, constipation and diarrhoea), frequent colds and any behavioural or learning problems, you should suspect a delayed food allergy and should have them tested to identify the culprit. The best test is IgG ELISA, which uses a finger-prick blood sample and a home test. Testing is best done under the guidance of a nutritional therapist or allergy expert (see Resources), who can devise a diet for your child that cuts out all allergy-provoking foods and includes suitable alternatives in order that the diet remains balanced and healthy. If more than a few foods are identified, this is an indicator of poor gut health, rather than multiple allergies, hence it is essential to address your child's gut health.

An alternative method of identifying food allergies is an elimination and challenge diet. This involves removing any likely culprits from your child's diet for a period of time (usually from two weeks to three months) and noting any changes in behaviour, and mental and physical symptoms. Then the foods can be reintroduced in a controlled way, while simultaneously monitoring your child's state of health. It has to be said, however, that this method has many shortcomings, because the range of foods a child can react to is so broad. Again, if you're making radical changes to what your child eats in order to follow an elimination and challenge diet, seek the advice of a qualified nutritional therapist to ensure that your child's diet remains balanced and healthy.

As you'll know if you or your child has an IgE allergy, the food in question, such as peanuts or shrimp, will probably have to be avoided for life, but IgG allergies, which have a relatively mild, delayed effect, may not be long-term. By identifying the foods that your child is allergic to, strictly avoiding them for around six months and improving their digestive health, your child may lose their allergy to them. However, in some cases, an IgG allergy reaction is, like an IgE allergy, for life. (See *Hidden Food Allergies* by Patrick Holford and Dr James Braly for more on this.)

## The gut factor

Digestive problems are often the underlying factor in a delayed-onset or IgG food allergy. Many children have excessively 'leaky' digestive tracts, which means that partially undigested proteins enter their bloodstream and trigger a reaction. The leakiness can develop with frequent use of antibiotics or aspirin, gastrointestinal infection or a deficiency in essential fats, vitamin A or zinc, so identifying and avoiding what your child is reacting to is just half the equation with an IgG food allergy. The other half is getting their digestion back into gear (see chapter 7 for more on this).

A child who has food allergy symptoms, such as frequent ear or chest infections, is likely to be prescribed antibiotics by their doctor. This can worsen gut health and worsen the allergy, leading in turn to more antibiotics and an unnecessary cycle of ill health. Clearly, it's best to deal with the root cause of the symptoms by identifying food allergens and removing them from your child's diet, rather than relying on antibiotics for short-term relief and thus perpetuating the problem in the long term.

## Summary

To test for, and reduce, your child's allergic potential:

- Completely remove wheat and dairy products from their diet for one month or more and see how they feel. In any case, try to limit these food groups in your child's diet by not including them in their diet every day.

- Improve your child's digestion by including plenty of fresh fruit, vegetables, seeds and fish in their diet, as these contain essential fats and zinc (see Chapter 7 for full details).

- Keep antibiotics to a minimum – they damage digestive health. Follow antibiotics with age-appropriate probiotics.

- If you suspect your child has a food allergy, have an IgG ELISA food allergy test and see a nutritional therapist, who can test what your child is allergic to, devise a course of action to reduce their allergic potential and ensure that your child's diet remains balanced and healthy while excluding the problem foods.

# Chapter 14

# Sniffles, wheezes, coughs and colds

Does your child just seem to be recovering from one infection when they come down with the next? Snotty noses, chest infections, ear infections, coughs, colds and asthma are standard fare for many children. If your child seems to lurch from one infection to the next, you need to look to the source and support their immune system.

We've already talked about the importance of gut health and its role in immunity, so if your child has frequent ear, nose and throat problems, start by completing the Digestion check and acting on the advice that follows it (see chapter 7).

## Asthma

The UK has one of the highest incidences of asthma in the world, with a whopping 5.2 million people currently receiving treatment for the condition. According to Asthma UK, one in ten – or 1.1 million – children has asthma.

Asthma is a condition that affects the airways – the small tubes that carry air in and out of the lungs. When a sufferer comes into contact with something that irritates their airways (an asthma trigger), the muscles around the walls of the airways tighten, so that the airways become narrower and the lining of the airways becomes inflamed and start to swell. Sometimes sticky mucus or phlegm builds up, which can further narrow the airways.

So why do children get asthma and why in increasing numbers? No one knows for sure, but there are a number of recognised risk factors. Children of parents with asthma, eczema or allergies are at higher risk. Environmental or lifestyle factors, such as increased pollution or, paradoxically, excessive hygiene, smoking in pregnancy and lack of breast-feeding also make children more susceptible. Some food additives are also linked with provoking asthma or may make asthma symptoms worse (see chapter 6 for details of additives to avoid).

Most children who are diagnosed with asthma will be expected to take asthma medication on a daily basis for many years, if not the rest of their life, but asthma medication is not without significant side-effects. However, by making a few simple changes to their diet, many children will be able to dispense with their medication altogether or to manage their symptoms with a lower dose.

## Magnesium magic

One of magnesium's many roles in the body is that of a muscle relaxant and by relaxing the lungs it can help prevent and treat acute asthma attacks. In a recent overview of studies published in the *Emergency Medicine Journal*, researchers undertook a systematic review of all the research on the use of magnesium for children requiring emergency treatment for an acute asthma attack. They found that magnesium given intravenously was highly beneficial in terms of improved lung function and a reduced need for hospitalisation.[1] Interestingly, children are frequently deficient in magnesium, so this treatment may work by simply addressing that deficiency.

Japanese researchers then went a step further and investigated whether asthma was related to a magnesium deficiency. In their study they measured magnesium levels in the red blood cells of stable asthma patients and also in a control group of people of a similar age who didn't have asthma. They found low magnesium levels in four out of ten of the asthmatics, compared with only one in ten of the controls.[2]

Magnesium's role in lung function was also studied by the Department of Preventive Medicine at UCLA, California. The team measured the lung function (flow and volume) of 2,566 children and compared this with their dietary intakes of magnesium, potassium and sodium. They found that the children with a low magnesium intake had worse lung function than those with a higher intake. Low potassium was also associated with poor lung function, but only in the girls.[3]

Magnesium is found in green, leafy vegetables and pumpkin seeds. Supplementation of between 50mg and 150mg is recommended for wheezy children.

## Antioxidants and fish

The same research team from UCLA, who looked at minerals and lung function above, also compared lung function and the intakes of antioxidant vitamins A, C and E from fruits, vegetables and juices for the same group of 2,566 children. This time they found lung function was poorer in the children, both boys and girls, who had the lowest intake of each of the three vitamins.[4]

Eating fish can also help children with asthma, as illustrated in a large study of the dietary habits of 20,271 European children aged seven to 11. The children who ate the least fish were 20 per cent more likely to have a persistent cough and 21 per cent more likely to wheeze. Those who ate the least summer fruit were 40 per cent more likely to have a winter cough and 35 per cent more likely to have a persistent cough.[5]

Similarly, a group of American researchers measured the intake of various antioxidant and anti-inflammatory foods and nutrients, including fruit, vegetables, vitamins C and E, beta-carotene, retinol (vitamin A) and omega-3 fatty acids, and compared these with the respiratory health of 2,112 eighteen-year-old high school students. The students who didn't eat much fruit had lower lung volume and were more likely to have chronic bronchitis, while those with the lowest omega-3 intake from oily fish were more likely to have chronic bronchitis, wheeze and asthma. Of the smokers, the worst symptoms were experienced by those with the lowest intake of vitamin C, suggesting that vitamin C has a protective effect against smoking.[6]

## Pollution

We're all well aware that smoking is bad for the lungs and there have been concerns about the effect of other forms of air pollution, such as exhaust fumes, on asthmatics. For example, in a study published in the *New England Journal of Medicine*, 60 adults with mild or moderate asthma walked for two hours along London's busiest shopping street, Oxford Street, and then on a separate occasion through the leafy, green expanse of Hyde Park. Lung function was worse in the asthmatics who spent two hours on Oxford Street and the Oxford Street walk also caused increased inflammation of their airways.[7]

Asthma may also be triggered by pollution inside your home. This primarily comes in the form of dust mites and pet hair. Reducing the places that these irritants can accumulate can improve your child's asthma. For example, you should remove carpets, have furnishings thoroughly cleaned, replace old feather pillows, vacuum regularly and put soft toys in the freezer periodically. Some children may be hypersensitive to common household chemicals such as room sprays and fabric deodorisers so these are best avoided.

Of course, it's nigh-on impossible to keep your child away from all air pollution, whether it's inside or beyond the home, so you must up their antioxidants and vitamin C for their protective effect.

# Blocked noses, colds and coughs

Ear, nose and throat symptoms are often caused by a combination of digestive problems and food allergies. If this sounds like your child, make sure they eat plenty of immune-boosting antioxidants from fresh fruits and vegetables, with lots of anti-inflammatory essential fats provided by oily fish, seeds and nuts (see chapter 7 for more on this).

## CASE HISTORY *Billy, age 14*

Billy's parents brought him to see us at the Brain Bio Centre. Billy had had mild asthma for years and it was being treated with the usual inhaled steroid medication. Of more concern to Billy's parents, however, was his constantly blocked and dripping nose, which meant he couldn't go anywhere without a tissue nor could he breathe through his nose. Sleeping was difficult and as a result he felt very tired at school. Billy also had some tell-tale digestive symptoms, including constipation, for which he needed regular laxatives. Tests revealed food allergies, so we strengthened his digestive system by temporarily excluding the culprit foods, and supplementing probiotics and glutamine powder. Within weeks, the nasal congestion eased, snoring reduced and Billy was sleeping better, which was reflected in better results in school.

## Vitamin C boost

When a child's immune system is fighting an infection, their requirement for vitamin C skyrockets. In fact, if they were a cat or a rat, a goat or a stoat, they would ramp up their own internal production of vitamin C to meet the additional need. Sadly, we primates lost the ability to manufacture vitamin C somewhere along our evolutionary journey, so we need to up our intake through food or supplements. During an active infection, give the amount of vitamin C we would usually recommend you supplement on a daily basis every two hours (see chapter 5 for more on this). Taken in excess, vitamin C causes loose bowels, so 'bowel tolerance' is a built-in alert that you've hit the upper level that the body requires. When bowel tolerance is reached and your child's stools become loose, drop the two-hourly dose by a third or so and maintain at that level (just below bowel tolerance) for a day or two. You'll find that a healthy child's bowel tolerance is at a much lower level than that of a child who's fighting an infection.

To treat a cough you might be inclined to use a cough syrup, but cough medicines don't work for children[8] and their popularity is probably due to their sedative effect, rather than anything else. What does work, though, is honey, which many cultures have used as an antiseptic for thousands of years. A recent study compared the effect of a single night-time dose of either honey, honey-flavoured cough syrup (containing dextromethorphan – a cough suppressant) or nothing on 105 children aged two to 18 who had a cough that was affecting their sleep. The honey was most effective in reducing cough frequency and severity, and improved the sleep quality of the children and their parents.[9]

Our favourite home remedy for coughs is a squeeze of lemon juice, a few slivers of ginger root and a teaspoon of honey in hot water, taken as a drink, although you must use good honey from a health food shop that retains its healthful properties, rather than heavily processed supermarket honey. Or try an ancient Ayurvedic remedy by taking half a teaspoon of fresh ginger juice (squeeze ginger root in a garlic press) and mixing it with a generous pinch of turmeric and a teaspoon of honey. Give one teaspoon morning and night or half a teaspoon for toddlers.

## To antibiotic or not to antibiotic...

Antibiotics were the usual treatment for a variety of childhood ailments until the rise of antibiotic resistance triggered a review of their use, and these days doctors are discouraged from treating infections with antibiotics until the infection has had a chance to resolve itself naturally. Ear infections, for example, are one of the most common childhood infections, but, painful as it might be for your child, most cases will clear up of their own accord.

Antibiotic use has been justified in the past as necessary to prevent chest, ear and throat infections developing into something more serious. However, in a recent study analysing the outcomes of 3.36 million episodes of such infections, it was found that the use of antibiotics was only justified to reduce the risk of serious complications for the elderly, not for children.[10]

The repeated use of antibiotics is damaging to gut health and therefore to immunity, so while they might help fight some bacterial infections in the short term, they weaken the immune system leaving your child at higher risk of further infections. Antibiotics do nothing for the 'common cold', which is a viral infection. If your child suffers with repeated chest, ear and throat infections we recommend you take a long-term view and focus on improving their diet and digestive health to strengthen their immunity.

## Summary

To reduce your child's susceptibility to ear, nose, throat and chest infections, and asthma:

- Optimise their gut health and investigate possible food allergies (see chapter 7 for more on this).

continues ➔

- Make sure their diet is rich in antioxidants, particularly if they are regularly exposed to air pollution.

- Optimise their intake of essential fats, especially omega-3 fats, by giving them flaxseeds, oily fish and/or fish oil supplements every day.

- Ensure a good intake of magnesium from green leafy vegetables and pumpkin seeds, particularly if they are prone to asthma. Consider supplementing an additional 50–150mg of magnesium daily for wheezing children.

- Ensure your home is free of irritants and allergens (see www.asthma.org.uk for more on this) and unnecessary chemicals.

- Ensure they avoid food additives that may worsen wheezing.

# Chapter 15

# The secrets of healthy skin

Skin. Where would we be without it? Not only does it keep our insides in, but it also protects us from infection, radiation and dehydration, keeps us warm and makes us look good. The entire surface of our bodies is replaced every 20 days and the degree to which the condition of our skin is influenced by what we eat and drink, as well as other factors such as our environment, is quite remarkable.

Skin is, after all, the largest organ in the body. In an adult it weighs around 5kg and has a surface area of 2m², about the size of a double bed. No other organ in the body is so exposed to external damage or disease, in the shape of injury, sunlight, environmental pollution and germs, yet at the same time our skin reflects many internal conditions and emotions, when it blushes or sweats, for example.

Similarly, some skin disorders, such as warts, are confined only to the skin, while others, indeed most of them, tell the story of what is going on inside. Cold sores and chicken pox show that the immune system is fighting off an internal infection, a rash may be the result of an allergic reaction to a food and a yellowish skin tone may indicate that there is a problem with the liver. All this tells us

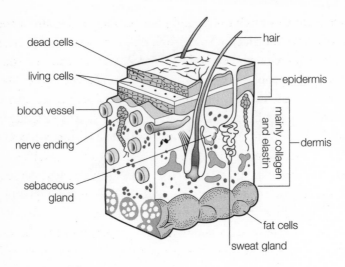

*A cross-section of skin*

that the condition of your child's skin is sensitive to a number of factors, including genes, hygiene, circulation, digestion, detoxification, immunity, the environment, psychological factors and, of course, what he or she eats.

Nutrition is fundamentally involved at every stage of skin development, starting with the inner layer of the skin, the dermis. This holds the main blood vessels and gives the body padding. It's principally made up of connective tissue and most of that connective tissue is made up of the protein collagen – vitamin C is essential in the production of collagen. Likewise, the protein keratin is a major component of skin, hair and nails and vitamin A is crucial in helping to control the rate of keratin accumulation in the skin. A lack of vitamin A can therefore result in dry, rough skin, while a diet rich in vitamin A can help to maintain healthy skin. The membranes of skin cells are made from essential fats and a lack of essential fats means these cells dry out too quickly, again resulting in dry skin.

The health of skin cells also depends on sufficient zinc, which is needed for the production of new generations of skin cells. Lack of zinc leads to stretch marks and poor healing, and is also associated with a wide variety of skin problems, from acne to eczema, so in many ways what you eat today you really do wear tomorrow.

Many skin problems can be traced to imbalances in the digestive system, including poor digestion and absorption, and an imbalance in gut flora, but if your child has skin problems, it's especially important that they limit their intake of sugar and saturated fat, and increase their intake of fresh fruit, vegetables and water. In particular, they need to eat plenty of antioxidant-rich foods every day. These include red, orange and yellow vegetables, and fruits such as sweet potatoes, carrots, apricots and watermelon, purple foods such as berries and grapes, green foods such as watercress, kale, alfalfa sprouts and broccoli, 'seed' foods such as peas and wholegrains, fresh nuts, seeds and their oils, and onions and garlic.

## A to Z of skin problems

### Acne

**Factors to consider**   Excess fat in the diet can mean the skin pores become blocked, leading to spots, plus vitamin A deficiency can mean too much keratin builds up in the skin, which again blocks the skin pores and leads to spots. Vitamin A and zinc deficiency also lead to a lowered ability to fight infection, as does lack of beneficial bacteria (often through over-use of antibiotics).

Zinc is particularly important in puberty and is likely to be especially low in teenage boys, as it's used for sperm production. If you spot white marks on your teenage son's fingernails, supplement 15mg of zinc.

**Diet**   Make sure it's low in fat and sugar, but high in water, seeds, oily fish, water-rich fresh fruit and vegetables. If skin doesn't respond to an improved diet, consider food allergies.

## Dermatitis

**Factors to consider**   Dermatitis literally means 'skin inflammation' and the term is used when the primary cause appears to be a contact allergy. The culprit could be the detergents in washing powders, soaps, shampoos or washing up liquid, the metals in jewellery or watches, the chemicals in perfumes and cosmetics. Where there is a contact allergy there is often a food allergy, too, commonly dairy products and wheat. Sometimes a combination of eating an allergy-provoking food and contact with an external allergen is needed for the symptoms to develop.

If your child isn't obtaining adequate essential fatty acids from oily fish and seeds, or consuming too much saturated fat or fried food, hormones called prostaglandins, which are formed from essential fatty acids and which control inflammation, won't function effectively.

One kind of dermatitis, called acrodermatitis, is primarily caused by zinc deficiency and responds exceptionally well to zinc supplementation.

**Diet**   Keep it low in saturated fat, and eat sufficient essential fats and very little meat or dairy produce. Test for a dairy or wheat allergy, if suspected, by avoiding these foods for a couple of weeks and seeing if there is any improvement. Switch to more natural detergents and cosmetics.

## Dry skin

**Factors to consider**   Slapping on moisturising cream certainly goes some way to relieving dry skin, but only some way. Without enough water each one of the cells in your child's body becomes dehydrated, losing its plumpness and structure, so the first step in keeping their skin well hydrated is to do just that – hydrate it by encouraging them to drink plenty of water every day. You can keep their skin well 'oiled' from the inside with essential fatty acids from oily fish, nuts and seeds. If your child has particularly dry skin, its worth supplementing them, too.

**Diet** This should be low in saturated fat and high in essential fatty acids from oily fish and seeds. Drink plenty of water every day, and eat plenty of water-rich fruit and vegetables.

## Eczema

**Factors to consider** As with dermatitis, the most common contributory factors are the combination of a food allergy (most often wheat or dairy) and a lack of essential fatty acids from oily fish and seeds, which have powerful anti-inflammatory effects.

**Diet** Make this low in saturated fat, which means low in meat and dairy, but sufficient essential fats from oily fish and seeds. Test for dairy and wheat allergy, if suspected, by avoiding these foods for a set period.

## Oily skin

**Factors to consider** As in the case of acne, excess fat in the diet can lead to greasiness, but puberty itself, and the hormonal changes that brings, can also be a factor.

**Diet** Ensure this contains sufficient essential fats from oily fish and seeds, but keep it low in fat and sugar.

## Psoriasis

**Factors to consider** Psoriasis is a completely different kind of skin condition to dermatitis or eczema and doesn't always respond as well to nutritional intervention, although it can occur when the body is 'toxic', perhaps due to digestive problems.

**Diet** Aim for a diet low in saturated fat, but with sufficient essential fats, low in meat and dairy produce, but high in fibre. Test for dairy and wheat allergy, if suspected, by avoiding these foods for a set period.

## Rashes

**Factors to consider** The root-causes of rashes can be difficult to pinpoint, but possible over-inflammation could be due to a lack of essential fatty acids, or food or contact allergy, or a viral, fungal or bacterial infection.

**Diet**    Again, make this low in saturated fat, but with sufficient essential fats, and low in meat and dairy produce. Test for dairy and wheat allergy, if suspected, by avoiding these foods for a set period.

## Summary

To ensure your child has good skin:

- Your child's diet should be rich in antioxidants, such as vitamins A, C, E and zinc. The best sources are fresh fruits, vegetables, oily fish and seeds.

- Plenty of water keeps the skin well hydrated.

- Excess saturated fat can make the skin oily and spotty, so limit if necessary.

- Reactive skin problems, such as dermatitis, eczema and rashes, may be related to food allergies, so test for these. Also, watch out for other irritants, such as soaps and cosmetics, and switch to 'natural' brands.

# Chapter 16

·

# Overcoming eating disorders

Anorexia and bulimia are complex and very serious conditions, and they are on the rise, but the good news is that they can be overcome. However, if your child has recently become much thinner, how can you know whether they are simply undereating and losing weight or have actually developed an eating disorder?

First off, anorexia is very rare in under-12s, as is bulimia – a condition involving binge eating followed by self-induced vomiting. If your child is under 12, their thinness could stem from an allergy or they may have developed a faddy attitude towards certain foods, perhaps egged on by their peers. If your child is 12 or older, though, it's possible that they are exhibiting signs of anorexia. That means it's important to know what eating disorders 'look like', so you can take appropriate action when and if you need to. The chart overleaf shows what to look out for.

## WHAT IS AN EATING DISORDER?

| Physical signs | Behavioural signs | Psychological signs |
| --- | --- | --- |
| **Anorexia nervosa** | **Anorexia nervosa** | **Anorexia nervosa** |
| • Severe weight loss | • Wanting to be left alone | • Intense fear of gaining weight |
| • Difficulty sleeping | • Wanting to have control | • Distorted perception of body weight and size |
| • Dizziness | • Wearing big, baggy clothes | • Obsession with dieting |
| • Stomach pains | • Excessive exercising | • Mood swings |
| • Constipation | • Difficulty concentrating | • Depressed |
| • Poor circulation and feeling cold | • Lying about eating meals | • Emotional |
| • Periods stop in women and girls | • Denying there is a problem | |
| • Hormonal changes in men and boys | | |
| **Bulimia** | **Bulimia** | **Bulimia** |
| • Sore throat or swollen glands | • Eating large quantities of food | • Ashamed |
| • Mouth infections | • Being sick after eating | • Guilty |
| • Sensitive or damaged teeth | • Being secretive | • Depressed |
| • Stomach pains | | • Mood swings |
| • Irregular periods | | • Feeling out of control |
| • Dry or poor skin | | |
| • Difficulty sleeping | | |
| **Binge eating** | **Binge eating** | **Binge eating** |
| • Weight gain | • Eating large quantities of food | • Emotional |
| | • Eating inappropriate food | • Depressed |
| | • Being secretive | • Mood swings |
| | | • Feeling out of control |

The underlying reasons for developing such severe and even life-threatening disorders can be extremely complicated. Many people with anorexia or bulimia have a problem or have been through a trauma that needs to be resolved with the help and support of a psychotherapist, but there are other possible strands to these difficult and puzzling conditions. Let's look at some of the latest research on nutritional links, which is leading to simple, pragmatic solutions that can work hand-in-hand with effective therapy.

## The zinc link

The idea that nutrition, or malnutrition, could play a part in the development and treatment of anorexia did not really emerge until the 1970s and 1980s, when scientists began to realise just how similar the symptoms and risk factors of anorexia and zinc deficiency were.[1-2] In fact, many risk factors in the two conditions are identical – both affect women under 25, and are linked to stress and puberty – and so are many of the symptoms, including:

- Weight loss
- Loss of appetite
- Amenorrhoea in women (periods stopping)
- Impotence in men
- Nausea
- Skin lesions
- Malabsorption of nutrients
- Depression
- Anxiety

## Confirming the connection

In 1980, the first trial studying zinc and anorexia started at the University of Kentucky in the US. The researchers discovered that ten out of 13 patients admitted with anorexia and eight out of 14 patients with bulimia were zinc-deficient on admission. Yet, after ample feeding, they became even more zinc-deficient. Since zinc is needed for the digestion and utilisation of protein, from which body tissue is made, the researchers recommended that extra zinc, above the amounts that would normally correct a deficiency, should be given to anorexics as they start to eat and gain weight.[3]

In 1984, the penny well and truly dropped with two important research findings. The first study showed that animals deprived of zinc very rapidly developed anorexic behaviour and loss of appetite, and that if these animals were force-fed a zinc-deficient diet to gain weight, they became seriously ill.[4] The second study showed that zinc deficiency damages the intestinal wall and therefore the absorption of nutrients, including zinc, potentially leading to a vicious spiral of deficiency.[5]

That same year, Professor Derek Bryce-Smith, now patron of the Institute for Optimum Nutrition, reported the first case of anorexia treated with zinc. The patient was a 13-year-old girl, tearful and depressed, weighing just 37kg. She was referred to a consultant psychiatrist, but, despite counselling, three months later her weight was 31.5kg. Then she began a course of zinc supplementation – 45mg a day. Within two months, she weighed 44.5kg, was cheerful again and had no significant zinc deficiency.[6]

In the mid-1980s, meanwhile, a trial with 15 anorexics began at the University of California. In 1987 the researchers reported: 'Zinc supplementation was followed by a decrease in depression and anxiety. Our data suggest that individuals with anorexia nervosa may be at risk for zinc deficiency and may respond favourably after zinc supplementation.'[7] By 1990, many researchers had found that over half of anorexic patients showed clear biochemical evidence of zinc deficiency.[8] Zinc supplementation couldn't be easier, but sadly, many treatment centres still fail to offer it.

## Chicken or egg?

The evidence linking zinc and anorexia is now beyond question. In fact, a recent review of all the research so far concludes: 'There is evidence that suggests zinc deficiency may be intimately involved with anorexia in humans: if not as an initiating cause, then as an accelerating or exacerbating factor that may deepen the pathology of anorexia.'[9] However, the fact that high levels of zinc supplementation help to treat anorexia does not mean that the cause of anorexia is zinc deficiency – it is psychological issues that usually trigger changes in the eating habits of susceptible people.

Anorexia can be a way of staving off adulthood and what are perceived as overwhelming fears and responsibilities. By avoiding eating, a young girl can repress the signs of growing up. Menstruation stops, breast size decreases and the body stays small. Starvation also induces a kind of 'high' by stimulating changes in important brain chemicals that may help to block out difficult feelings and issues that are too hard to face.

So where does zinc come in? Many anorexics choose to become vegetarian, and most vegetarian diets are lower in zinc, essential fats and protein, according to a study at the Health Sciences Department of the British Columbia Institute of Technology in Burnaby, Canada, which analysed the diets of vegetarian anorexics, versus non-vegetarian patients.[10]

Whether vegetarian or not, once the pattern of not eating is chosen and becomes established, zinc deficiency is almost inevitable, due both to poor intake and poor absorption. With it comes a further loss of appetite and further depression, along with an inability to cope with the stresses that face many adolescents growing up in the 21st century.

The optimum nutrition approach to helping someone with anorexia or bulimia is best adopted alongside sessions with a skilled psychotherapist. The nutritional approach emphasises quality of food rather than quantity, plus supplements, which would almost certainly include 45mg of zinc a day, reducing to half that once weight gain is achieved and maintained.

## Tryptophan and appetite

A loss of weight and muscle tissue indicates protein deficiency. Obviously, anorexia or bulimia sufferers are unlikely to be getting enough protein or they may have trouble digesting, absorbing or metabolising it. The amino acids valine, isoleucine and tryptophan have been found to be low in people with anorexia, and supplementing valine and isoleucine helps to build muscle, while tryptophan is the building block of serotonin, which controls both mood and appetite.

Recent research has found striking differences in the blood levels of tryptophan in people with anorexia,[11] and both starvation and excessive exercise have emerged as factors in these levels.[12] So far, the evidence points to problems with how anorexics or bulimics respond to low levels of tryptophan. As the conversion of tryptophan into serotonin is both zinc- and B6-dependent, all three nutrients may be needed for proper appetite control, as well as a balanced, happy mood.

The interplay between body and mind, or nutrients and behaviour, is well illustrated by recent research at Oxford University's psychiatry department by Dr Philip Cowen and colleagues. Cowen and his team found, not surprisingly, that levels of tryptophan and serotonin were lower in women on calorie-restricted diets. They also found, however, that recovered bulimics put on a diet free of tryptophan rapidly become more depressed, and overly concerned about their weight and shape, as well as more fearful of losing control over their eating.[13]

Looked at together, all this research strongly suggests that people prone to anorexia or bulimia have a special need for tryptophan, and probably zinc and B6, and that when deprived of these nutrients they are more likely to develop unhealthy responses to stress, such as the loss of appetite control.

The most direct way of addressing these imbalances in people with eating disorders is to supplement tryptophan, or 5-hydroxytryptophan (5-HTP), plus zinc and B6. In the long run, however, the goal has got to be a change in diet. Often, especially in anorexics, supplements such as concentrated fish oils are easier to handle at the start because, unlike food, they contain virtually no calories. As the person's nutritional status improves, their anxieties and obsessive/compulsive tendencies reduce, and they almost always see the logic of making positive dietary changes.

The ideal diet should include foods that are easy to eat and digest, as well as being highly nutritious. Good quality protein such as quinoa, fish, soya and spirulina or blue-green algae is important, as are ground seeds, lentils, beans, fruits and vegetables.

Fish and seeds are especially important, because they contain essential fats. Since most people with eating disorders go out of their way to avoid fat, their diets are frequently low in these essential nutrients, which, as we've seen, really are essential when it comes to mental health. Also, essential fats are vital for both making serotonin and receiving the serotonin signals that cross from one neuron to another – in other words, for spreading the happiness around.

## Pinning down binge foods

The foods people with bulimia binge on tend to reveal that they have food sensitivities or blood sugar problems. The most common binge foods are sweet, wheat-based or dairy products. Both wheat and dairy products contain exorphins, chemicals that mimic (and can therefore block) pleasure-giving endorphins in the brain and may therefore influence behaviour. What's more, when a bulimic's blood sugar is very low – as it would be after a fast or vomiting – they would inevitably crave sweet foods for a quick sugar fix.

The effects of all these foods can contribute to the erratic or compulsive behaviour of people struggling with bulimia. We often ask people with bulimia to binge as much as they like for the next two weeks, but not on any of these foods. Many of them report that their desire to binge at all is dramatically reduced immediately.

Don't think, however, that if your child is, say, more prone to react strongly to the lack of a nutrient like zinc or tryptophan, that that's the whole story. As we have said, biochemistry does not exclude psychological problems as part of the reason your child has developed an eating disorder, so seek constructive help from a sensitive and reliable therapist.

## Summary

To support your child if they are dealing with an eating disorder:

- See a nutritional therapist who can assess what your child is deficient in and advise you accordingly.

- Their advice will probably include supplementing zinc, 5-HTP, B6, plus essential fats, either in capsules or in seeds and fish.

- Take your child to see a psychotherapist with experience of helping children with eating disorders to make a full recovery.

## Chapter 17

·

# Curing sleep problems

Can't sleep, won't sleep? One of the most common problems parents face is children who have difficulty sleeping and the result isn't just mentally exhausted children who struggle to learn, concentrate and behave, but parents who exist in a permanent state of tiredness themselves. Research showed many years ago that one key to growth and development in children is a good night's sleep, so poor sleep delivers a double whammy – a short-term impact on your child's performance, energy and mood, and an insidious curb on their development that could prevent them from reaching their full potential as an older child and adult.

### CASE HISTORY *James, age seven*

James' mother brought him to see us at the Brain Bio Centre because, no matter how tired he became, he simply was not sleeping. Consequently, his concentration and memory at school were very poor. We screened him for various biochemical imbalances and analysed his diet. We found that James had food allergies, low levels of calcium and magnesium, and too much sugar in his diet. By excluding the foods that James was allergic to, reducing his sugar intake and supplementing extra calcium and magnesium, James' sleep improved significantly within a matter of weeks.

## Is your child sleep-deprived?

School-aged children need something between nine and 12 hours of sleep at night, but it's easy to tell if they're getting enough – they go to bed, fall asleep easily, wake up easily and are never tired during the day.

Without sleep, even for a night, the body shows clear signs of stress – mood and concentration go, defences drop, zinc and magnesium levels fall, and vitamin C is used up at an alarming rate. Sleep rejuvenates both body and mind. In fact, during the first three hours of sleep, the body goes into rapid repair mode.

Sleep specialists at Loughborough University in the UK have carried out tests into how the brain functions when it is deprived of sleep and, as you might expect, sleepy people have problems finding the right words, coming up with ideas and coping with rapidly changing situations.[1] Sleep deprivation makes us moody and irritable, and, in the long term, even depressed. When it's tired, the body also finds it harder to fight off infections.[2]

There are two main types of sleep problems – trouble getting to sleep and trouble staying asleep. If your child resists going to bed and kicks up a fuss every night at bedtime, it could be that he or she faces the inevitable prospect of lying awake for hours feeling bored and frustrated before they finally drop off. However, a television, games console or computer in the bedroom is not the answer, since research shows that these make sleep problems even worse.[3]

## Finding the zzzzz factor

Whichever type of sleep problem your child has, the factors to consider are the same: along with habitual telly-gazing last thing at night, these include deficiencies of the calming minerals magnesium and calcium, excess sugar or stimulants, food allergies and a lack of physical activity during the day.

## Chill-out minerals

If your child fails to get enough magnesium and calcium, it can trigger or exacerbate sleep difficulties, because this mineral duo calms the body, and helps relax nerves and muscles. As we've seen, magnesium deficiency is increasingly common in children. In fact, your child's diet is likely to be lower in magnesium than in calcium, so make sure they're eating plenty of magnesium-rich foods – seeds, nuts, green vegetables, wholegrains and seafood. Including some magnesium in the evening, perhaps even in a supplement, may help. If your breast-fed baby is having trouble sleeping, you can take a magnesium supplement yourself and your baby will receive it through your milk. Particularly good sources of calcium, meanwhile, include milk products, green vegetables, nuts, seafood and molasses.

Other nutrients that are important for good sleep are the B vitamins. These are best taken earlier in the day rather than in the evening, though, as they are also involved in energy production and can be overstimulating just before bed.

## Cutting out stress, sugar and stimulants

Many of the daily rhythms in your child's body, including those dictating energy and sleepiness, are finely tuned mechanisms that depend on certain hormonal patterns, chemicals and nutrients. At night, the levels of the stress hormone cortisol should dip, calming your child down and preparing the body for sleep. If, however, their cortisol levels are out of kilter for any reason (usually due to stress or a diet high in stimulants or sugar), their ability to get to sleep, to sleep through the night or to wake up refreshed is likely to be impaired.

If cortisol levels are high at night, for instance, this suppresses the release of growth hormones, which are essential for daily tissue repair and growth. Consequently, it's an excellent idea to establish a 20- to 30-minute nightly 'calm-down' bedtime routine, which can include taking a bath, putting on pyjamas, reading and other relaxing activities.

Many parents whose children wake in the night and then can't get back to sleep find that, once they start keeping their blood sugar levels even during the day, it sets the scene for the correct patterns at night, giving them more chance of a good night's sleep. A light, low-GL snack half an hour to an hour before bed ensures not only that your child is not kept awake by hunger pangs, but also that he or she won't be woken during the night by a drop in blood sugar levels. A small piece of fruit and a handful of seeds or a couple of oatcakes and some nut butter are ideal. Caffeine – and this includes chocolate – should be avoided entirely. Even small amounts taken early in the day can keep children awake at night.

## Solving sleep apnoea

Children who have a chronically blocked nose may suffer from sleep apnoea, a condition usually associated with older adults. In sleep apnoea, your sleeping child will struggle to breathe to the point of waking up, or at least will have a very restless night. If your child has a stuffy or runny nose and is a 'mouth-breather', you should suspect food allergies (see chapter 13 for more on this).

## Serotonin and melatonin

The amounts of serotonin and the hormone melatonin in our bodies increase in the evening as part of our natural sleep–wake cycle. Deficiencies in either can prevent sleep and disruptions in sleep patterns can deplete the body of these substances.

The body needs adequate amounts of B6 and tryptophan to make serotonin and melatonin, and foods particularly high in tryptophan include chicken, cheese, tuna, tofu, eggs, nuts, seeds and milk. So, as so often happens, a traditional remedy – drinking a glass of milk before bed – makes scientific sense. (Other foods associated with inducing sleep are lettuce, which contains a substance related to opium, and oats.)

The amino acid our bodies use to make serotonin and melatonin is 5-HTP, so supplementing 5-HTP for a month can be useful as a way of normalising sleep patterns, once all the other obstacles to sleep have been addressed. When your child is sleeping well again, they can stop taking the supplements. We recommend 25mg an hour before bed for children under eight and 50mg for older children.

Melatonin production in the body is lowered by bright light, so make sure all the lights in your child's bedroom are dimmed before they go to sleep. Incidentally, for their visual development it's best that they sleep in a dark room, so don't use a night light unnecessarily. You can get up to 100mcg of melatonin, a tenth of 1mg (an adult supplement dose is between 1mg and 10mg daily), in an 85g serving of oats, brown rice or sweetcorn. Bananas and tomatoes have half this amount, so serving these foods in the evening may help your child sleep.

Melatonin is a neurotransmitter, not a nutrient, and hence needs to be used much more cautiously when supplementing. Taking too much can cause diarrhoea, constipation, nausea, dizziness, headaches, depression and nightmares. However, melatonin has been used to good effect in children in a number of studies,[4] so it's worth a try under the guidance of a qualified nutritional therapist or doctor. Melatonin cannot be bought over the counter in Britain, but is available by mail order or on the web from the US.

## Running out the restlessness

Ever watched your child tearing around a playground and thought, 'They'll sleep well tonight'? It's true. Exercise de-stresses, and promotes calmness and a sense of well-being, partly through the release of endorphins. So aside from PE at school, encourage your child to get active at weekends and in the afternoon, rather than simply slumping in front of the TV or computer. They're sure to find something they enjoy – swimming, football with friends, tennis, dance class, or just a brisk walk in the park or a spin on their bike. Just ensure they don't exercise too late in the evening, as the energising effects of all that activity may promote sleeplessness.

## Summary

To ensure your child get a good night's sleep:

- Avoid sugar and stimulants, especially after 4pm.

- Follow a regular, calming bedtime routine every evening.

- Supplement magnesium and calcium in the evening, and ensure your child eats plenty of magnesium and calcium-rich foods, such as seeds and crunchy or dark green vegetables.

- To re-establish a good sleep pattern, try 10 to 25mg of 5-HTP and perhaps melatonin under supervision.

- Limit television to no more than two hours a day and, if there is a television, computer or games console in your child's bedroom, remove it.

- Ensure your child has plenty of stimulating physical activity during the day, so they are ready for sleep in the evening.

# Chapter 18

.

# Enhancing mood and behaviour

Childhood is supposed to be a joyful time, but it doesn't always pan out that way and many children are no strangers to sadness, boredom, irritability and anger. Since 2004, there has been a virtual ban in the UK on prescribing antidepressants for children, in recognition of their ineffectiveness and the increased risk of suicide associated with them, among other side-effects. However, there are much better solutions than this to hand, so if your child cries a lot, doesn't enjoy or participate in activities, has low self-esteem, is hostile to others or is self-destructive, you can help them. There are two avenues to explore – psychological and biochemical – but, as we'll see, they're intimately intertwined.

## Getting to the root of unhappiness

Conventionally, anger is not an emotion we, much less children, are allowed to express. Some children – angry at something that has happened at school, with their friends or at home – bottle it up as depression. Although you, as a parent, can help tremendously, every child also benefits from having an open, sympathetic adult other than their parents to talk to and to help them find solutions to their problems. The UK charity Childline, for instance, receives around 2,000 calls each year from children who are distressed and desperate.

One of the greatest unrecognised truths is the role of nutrition in the psychological health of our children. Ensuring your child is optimally nourished will not only improve their mood, but also give them the energy and motivation to deal with life's inevitable ups and downs. Few child psychotherapists and paediatricians recognise how much better their results would be if they helped children tune up their brain biochemistry.

There are a number of common imbalances connected to nutrition that can worsen a child's mood and motivation, some of which you will already be familiar with:

**Factors with a negative effect on mood**

- Blood sugar imbalances (often associated with excessive sugar and caffeine intake)

- Nutrient deficiencies (vitamin B3, B6, B12, C, folic acid, zinc, magnesium and essential fats)

- Tryptophan and tyrosine deficiencies (a lack of the substances that help build neurotransmitters)

- Allergies and sensitivities

Poor control of blood glucose levels is a huge factor in low mood, yet a relatively simple aspect of your child's daily routine to fix. As we saw in chapter 2, you can help them here by always providing breakfast, as well as regular meals and snacks composed of natural, unprocessed foods, but what about those key nutrients?

## Beating the blues with nutrition

Among nutrients, the most promising for improving mood are vitamins B3, B12 and folic acid, then vitamin B6, zinc and magnesium and the essential fats, especially omega-3s (see chapter 3 for more on this).

Folic acid is found in green leafy vegetables, nuts, seeds and beans. Far too many children have far too few of these, yet their effect can be astounding. Folic acid and other B vitamins are involved in the biochemical process known as methylation, which is critical for balancing the neurotransmitters that keep your child motivated and happy.

Zinc and magnesium are among the most important minerals for mental health. We've seen how zinc, for instance, helps with problems such as confusion, depression and slow mental processing. Magnesium relaxes both the mind and muscles, and deficiencies are very common, manifesting as muscle aches, cramps and spasms, as well an anxiety, irritability and insomnia. Children often have low levels of magnesium, which can be helped via supplementation. Seeds and nuts are rich in magnesium, as are vegetables and fruit, especially dark green leafy vegetables, such as kale or spinach. We recommend that children eat these magnesium-rich foods every day and supplement an additional 50 to 100mg of magnesium.

## Fats to fight depression

We've already encountered omega-3 fish oils in a number of contexts and they are very much part of the equation for happiness, too. The better a child's blood levels of omega-3 fats, the better their levels of serotonin – the 'happy' neurotransmitter – are likely to be. The reason for this is that omega-3 fats help build the brain's receptor sites for serotonin, as well as improving reception. According to Dr Joseph Hibbeln, who discovered that fish eaters are less prone to depression, 'It's like building more serotonin factories, instead of just increasing the efficiency of the serotonin you have.'[1] Many trials have now been published proving that omega-3 fats are highly effective as a treatment for depression and[2] EPA is the top omega-3 for this job.

A case in point is a small-scale study by Professor Basant Puri from London's Hammersmith Hospital. Puri decided to try ethyl-EPA on one of his patients, a 21-year-old student who had been on a variety of antidepressants, to no avail. He had very low self-esteem, sleeping problems, little appetite, found it hard to socialise and often thought of killing himself. After a month of supplementing omega-3 fats, he was no longer having suicidal thoughts and after nine months his depression had disappeared.[3]

## Neurotransmitters and mood – a balancing act

There are often two sides to feeling low – feeling miserable and feeling apathetic. The most prevalent theory for the cause of these imbalances is a brain imbalance in two families of neurotransmitters. These are serotonin, which influences your mood, and adrenalin and noradrenalin, which influence your motivation. However, this imbalance isn't just about nutrition, so let's look at some of the other factors in your child's life that could be fuelling any unhappiness and apathy they're experiencing.

### Stresses and strains – how imbalance sets in

The mad, goal-driven dash of 21st-century living can be very stressful for children. Too many children are pressured to perform in a century where the motto is 'succeed and achieve'. Perhaps living out their parents' dissatisfactions, they go from school to piano lessons to extra coaching, with no time left to simply play, dream or do nothing.

All this has an inevitable effect on the brain, which produces more and more adrenalin and serotonin in response to the too frequent ups and downs, and numerous stresses and strains. It's akin to the body's production of more and more insulin to even out frequently fluctuating blood sugar levels. This increases a child's need for the building blocks, the amino acids, from which we make these mood-enhancing neurotransmitters. Combine these psychological pressures with a poor diet and too many children go over the edge into low moods and erratic behaviour.

Over the last few years, what has been learnt about both serotonin, the 'happy' neurotransmitter, and adrenalin and noradrenalin, 'the motivators', is that there are four main reasons for deficiency in children, in addition to a lack of amino acids. These are:

- Not enough light

- Not enough exercise

- Too much stress

- Not enough B vitamins, zinc and magnesium

So if your child is melancholy or depressed, misbehaving, exhausted, tends to comfort-eat and has disturbed sleep patterns, the chances are that a combination of factors are working together to leave them short on serotonin, adrenalin or noradrenalin.

How does it happen? Light is very important as a brain stimulator, yet with our increasingly indoor lives most of us don't get enough of it. The difference in light exposure outside and inside is massive. Many of us spend 23 out of 24 hours a day indoors, exposed to an average of 100 units (called lux) of light. Compare that to the 20,000 lux of a sunny day and 7,000 lux of an overcast day. Most of us are simply not exposing ourselves to enough direct sunlight to maximise serotonin production and, of course, it's worse in winter when the days are shorter.

Vitamin D, the sunshine vitamin, can become deficient in winter, too. It's an important mood-boosting vitamin and low levels are linked with seasonal affective disorder (SAD), a form of 'winter blues'. Most of our vitamin D is made in the skin in sunlight, but there are small amounts in oily fish, milk and eggs. If you're not able to jet off for some winter sunshine, then a daily supplement of between 3 to 12mcg, depending on age, is recommended.

Stress – say, from exams or bullying – rapidly reduces serotonin levels and also raises adrenalin, leading to burnout. A couch-potato habit can make this worse, because physical exercise improves the stress response and reduces the stress-induced depletion of serotonin and adrenalin.

Exercise itself is an incredibly powerful mood booster. When 202 adults with 'major depression' were given either an antidepressant drug, a placebo pill or an exercise programme for four months by a research team at Duke University Medical Center in the US, the exercise was as effective at lifting mood as the medication.[4] The message is that you need to ensure your child has the time and opportunity to play outdoors for a reasonable amount of time each day, and get daily exercise.

## Supplementing for neurotransmitter balance

You might find that your child needs extra help in recovering from difficulties with mood. In these cases, you should look to supplementation and there are a number of possibilities.

### Go for the right amino acids

Serotonin is made from a constituent of protein, the amino acid tryptophan. Dr Philip Cowen from Oxford University's psychiatry department has proven that if you deprive adults of tryptophan, most experience a worsening of mood and start to show signs of depression within seven hours.[5] Tryptophan is especially abundant in fish, turkey, chicken, cheese, beans, tofu, oats and eggs. A child's diet, depending on age, needs to contain between 500mg and 1,000mg of tryptophan a day, which they can easily achieve by eating one or two of the following meals, each providing 500mg of it:

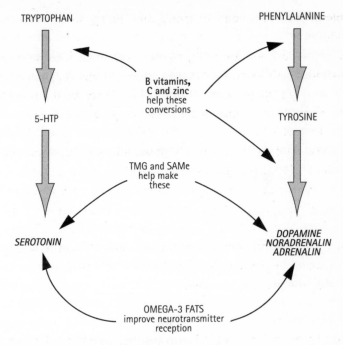

*How nutrients affect mood-boosting neurotransmitters*

- Oat porridge, soya milk and two scrambled eggs
- Baked potato with cottage cheese and tuna salad
- Chicken breast, potatoes au gratin and green beans
- Wholewheat spaghetti with bean, tofu or meat sauce
- Salmon fillet, quinoa and lentil pilaf, and green salad with yoghurt dressing.

Adrenalin and noradrenalin are made from the food amino acids called phenylalanine and tyrosine. These are also found in protein foods – the same kind that are rich in tryptophan – so, as we saw in chapter 4, ensuring adequate protein intake helps keep your child's mood and motivation positive.

In adult studies, supplementing 5-HTP, the amino acid from which the body makes serotonin, along with tyrosine, the amino acid from which the body makes adrenalin and noradrenalin, has proven highly effective in correcting mood problems. Not only is 5-HTP an efficient mood-booster, much more so than antidepressants, it also has no significant side-effects[6] and the worst that seems to happen is that, in very large doses, some people become nauseated. For children, depending on age, supplement between 20 and 50mg 5-HTP.

## Try TMG – the master tuner

In the diagram on the previous page, showing how nutrients affect mood-boosting neurotransmitters, you may have noticed two unfamiliar, strange-sounding nutrients. TMG (tri-methylglycine) and SAMe (s-adenosyl methionine) are both amino acids that play an important role in the process called methylation, which helps form most neurotransmitters (see chapter 8 for more on this).

This trio, B6, B12 and folic acid, control a critical process in the body called methylation, which is vital in the formation of almost all neurotransmitters. Abnormal methylation lies behind many health problems. These three are also key to managing the levels of an amino acid called homocysteine. Elevated levels of homocysteine have been linked to an increased risk of, among others diseases, cardiovascular problems and osteoporosis.

SAMe is one of the most comprehensively studied natural anti-depressants. Over 100 studies show that SAMe is equal to or superior to antidepressants, and works faster – most often within a few days (most pharmaceutical antidepressants may take three to six weeks to take effect), and with few side-effects.[7–8]

While SAMe is classified as a medicine, TMG, the amino acid from which it is made, is a component of food, and is especially high in roots and sprouts. So eating carrots, parsnips, beetroot, turnip, swedes, potato and beansprouts will provide your child with TMG. Although it's not classified as an essential nutrient, we recommend that children eat at least 100mg a day, which translates into one serving of a root vegetable or sprout.

To help children with behavioural problems and low mood, give them supplements containing all these amino acids (5-HTP, phenylalanine or tyrosine and TMG) together with the B vitamins that help turn them into neurotransmitters (B3, B6, B12 and folic acid). Some children's formulas contain these nutrients, which literally help the brain to make connections.

At the Brain Bio Centre, we analyse children's blood and test for things such as essential fats, vitamin D and the amino acid homocysteine, the indicator of vitamin B deficiency associated with low academic achievement. Given this information, we can devise the perfect nutrition programme of food and supplements to help them achieve their full potential.

## CASE HISTORY *Liam, age 14*

Liam was treated at the Brain Bio Centre having been excluded from mainstream school for disruptive behaviour. We tested him and found that his homocysteine score was 24 – the average for a 90-year-old! We put him on a low-sugar diet and supplemented B vitamins, magnesium, TMG and omega-3. One month later his homocycsteine score was down to nine. He told us, 'About ten days after starting the diet and the vitamins I noticed I was less tired in the morning. Now I'm not tired at all when I wake up. I have loads more energy, I'm less bored and I feel a lot happier. I'm getting on better at school and concentrating better in class. I'm also doing more activities and sports. I'm now a lot calmer than I used to be, I haven't got into trouble at all and I feel more positive about my future. I'm going to stay on the diet for life and keep taking the vitamins. It's brilliant!'

# Addressing aggression

Has your child ever lashed out uncontrollably and violently towards you or someone else? It's a huge shock and, what's more, can be completely mystifying, but be assured that you're not alone. At the Brain Bio Centre, we see many cases of children, some very young, who are uncontrollable, violent and show no apparent remorse for their actions. Sadly, the problem grows with the child, so if it isn't addressed it's almost certainly going to get worse as they approach adulthood.

This scenario, however, is in no way inevitable. You've already have seen how today's unbalanced, unhealthy diet affects the brain and, true to form, we find that the major contributors to aggressive behaviour are the usual suspects – too much sugar, not enough essential fats, food allergies and brain pollution.

## CASE HISTORY *Charles, age eight*

Charles' parents brought him to see us at the Brain bio Centre, because they were concerned about his very aggressive and violent behaviour. Tests revealed food allergies, a homocysteine score of 14 and elevated aluminium in his hair. We recommended a specific supplement designed to reduce his homocysteine levels and to help his body detoxify the aluminium. We also suggested he avoided the foods that he was allergic to. After ten weeks, his parents reported that he was much more focused, calmer and rational, and wasn't lashing out like he had been. He had also stopped wetting himself, which had been a problem before.

As we have seen, all thoughts and consequently all behaviour are processed through the brain and nervous system, which are – like the rest of the body – completely dependent on nutrition to keep them functioning. It's astonishing, but approximately half of all the glucose in the blood goes to power the brain, which is also dependent on a second-by-second supply of micronutrients – vitamins, minerals and essential fats. Meanwhile, any anti-nutrients in your child's body, such as cadmium and lead, will fundamentally affect brain function.

To date, there has been very little research into the effects of altering the diet of small children with aggression problems. However, there have been some excellent studies in adolescents, showing dramatic reductions in violent behaviour over a short space of time just by giving them small amounts of essential nutrients.

## Calming aggressive behaviour

We feel there is much you can do to help your child nutritionally if they're often overcome with feelings of anger or engage in aggressive behaviour. Let's look at some of the options.

### Sorting out sugar-fuelled fury

The involvement of blood sugar fluctuations in behaviour is an intimate one. A 'rebound low', otherwise known as reactive hypoglycaemia, can occur when a child consumes sugar, refined carbs or stimulants. The rapid rise in blood sugar levels can be followed by a crash, resulting in extreme tiredness, irritability, depression and aggression. In addition, if a child feels this bad, they're much more likely to behave badly, because exhaustion leads to poor impulse control. If your child's behaviour is volatile and out of control, getting to grips with any blood sugar problems is vital (see chapter 2 for more on this).

### Omegas – how to calm hostility

A deficiency in essential fats is increasingly being seen as a real contributor to aberrant behaviour. Changes in modern diets have certainly reduced our intake of these essential fats and, as we've seen, if the mother is deficient during pregnancy, it could have long-lasting effects on the child's mental development and behaviour.

Recent research by Dr Tomohito Hamazaki of Toyama University in Japan suggests that omega-3 fats help control anger and hostility. He reasoned that under conditions of stress a certain level of aggression could have survival value, but, from an evolutionary point of view, too much aggression would have the opposite effect. He therefore decided to see what would happen if he gave omega-3 fats to students taking exams. He gave them 1.5g of DHA, or a placebo, and measured their hostility using psychological tests at the start of the study and again three months later. The second test, which was administered just before the exams, showed a 59 per cent jump in hostile reactions in those taking the placebo, but no change at all in the students taking the omega-3 fats.[9] Omega-3 fats, it seems, help children to keep their heads in stressful situations.

## Countering nutritional deficiencies

Essential fats aren't the only key to calmer behaviour, though, and deficiencies in calcium, magnesium, zinc and selenium have all been shown to correlate with increases in violence.

The simple addition of a multivitamin and mineral supplement containing RDA levels of nutrients has been shown to have extremely positive effects on behaviour in prison populations in the US, according to extensive research by Dr Stephen Schoenthaler of the Department of Social and Criminal Justice at California State University, Stanislaus, whose work we looked at earlier. In a recent study, Schoenthaler compared the behaviour of young offenders in the three months prior to and during supplementation, versus the behaviour of those given a placebo. There was an overall reduction in recorded offences of 40 per cent, with the subjects on supplements producing 22 per cent fewer assaults on staff and a 21 per cent reduction in violent and non-violent antisocial behaviour compared with the subjects on the placebo.

Blood tests for vitamins and minerals showed that around a third of the offenders had low levels of one or more vitamins and minerals before the trial. Those whose levels had become normal by the end of the study demonstrated a massive improvement in behaviour of between 70 and 90 per cent.[10] We believe it's not rocket science to make the leap that if adequate levels of these nutrients can have such dramatic effects on these adolescents, they will also help younger children with aggressive behaviour.

## Antisocial foods

Severe allergic reactions can produce dramatic changes in behaviour, as has been well reported in hyperactive children who have chemical or food intolerances,[11] as well as in young offenders[12] (see chapter 13 for more on this).

# Bipolar children

Some children with aggression problems have bipolar disorder – the condition formerly known as manic depression – and may oscillate from states of mania and hyperactivity to crying and depression. The trouble is, though, that bipolar disorder simply isn't diagnosed in childhood. In fact, it used to be thought that it didn't exist in the under-20s, but this just isn't true.

Bipolar disorder can and does occur in infancy, but the majority of the children who have it are wrongly classified as having ADHD. Doctors Janet Wozniak and Joseph Biederman from Harvard Medical School found that 94 per cent of children with mania also met the criteria for a diagnosis of ADHD. This is bad news, because the last thing a child with bipolar disorder needs is stimulant drugs such as Ritalin.

Dr Demitri Papalos, associate professor of psychiatry at Albert

Einstein College of Medicine in New York City, studied the effects of stimulant drugs on 73 children diagnosed as bipolar. Disturbingly, he found that 47 of these children were thrown into states of mania or psychosis by stimulant medication.[13] His excellent book, *The Bipolar Child*, co-authored with his wife Janice Papalos, helps to differentiate between children suffering from bipolar disorder and children with ADHD.

These are the characteristics and differences they've observed:

- Children with bipolar disorder essentially have a mood disorder and go from extreme highs, with mania, tantrums and anger, to extreme lows. Some may go through four cycles in a year, others may have week-long cycles. This rapid cycling is rarely seen in adults.

- Bipolar children also have different kinds of angry outbursts. While most children will calm down in 20 to 30 minutes, bipolar children can rage on for hours, often with destructive, even sadistic, aggressiveness. During an angry outburst they can also display disorganised thinking, language and body positions.

- Bipolar children have bouts of depression, which is not a usual pattern of ADHD. Many show giftedness, perhaps in verbal or artistic skills, often early in life. Their misbehaviour is often more intentional, while the classic ADHD child often misbehaves through being inattentive. A bipolar child can, for example, be the bully in the playground.

Our nutritional approach is likely to be helpful for children with bipolar disorder. Ritalin and other stimulant drugs can be an absolute disaster.

## Summary

To keep your child's mood, motivation and behaviour good:

- Give them a diet containing protein-rich foods (fish, meat, eggs, pulses) and TMG-rich foods (root vegetables and sprouts).

- Optimise your child's intake of essential fats, especially omega-3 fats, by giving them flaxseeds, oily fish and/or fish oil supplements every day.

- Ensure optimum nutrition with a good multivitamin that provides all the B vitamins, plus magnesium and zinc.

- If your child is low in energy, mood or motivation, or is under stress, underperforming or acting up, give them an additional supplement containing TMG, 5-HTP, tyrosine or phenylalanine.

- Ensure your child gets regular exercise and sunshine to boost their mood and vitamin D.

- Remove sugar and additives from their diet, and check for food allergies.

- Depression and aggression are psychological, as well as nutritional issues and you may find you need to follow a complementary approach. Alongside the methods suggested here, consider finding a therapist to address any psychological or family dynamic issues.

# Chapter 19

·

# Drug-free solutions for ADHD

Nowadays, any child with learning and behavioural problems tends to get put into one of a number of boxes. Are they dyslexic, because they're having problems with words and writing? Are they dyspraxic, because they're having problems with coordination? Do they have ADHD, the official term for what used to be known as hyperactivity, but which still denotes poor attention span, concentration and hyperactive behaviour?

In most children who have problems with learning or behaviour, there are substantial overlaps between these categories. While a minority of children are purely dyslexic, more will show features of two, three or all of these conditions in differing degrees of severity. Around half the dyslexic population is likely to be dyspraxic and vice versa, and the mutual overlap between ADHD and dyslexia/dyspraxia is also around 50 per cent.[1] Unfortunately, though, it's rare to find a diagnosis or treatment that takes account of these complexities. ADHD, for instance, lies firmly in the realm of psychiatry and is usually treated with stimulant medication.

Current evidence suggests that up to 20 per cent of the population may be affected to some degree by one or more of these conditions and the associated difficulties usually persist into adulthood, causing serious problems not only for those affected, but for society as a whole. It seems incredible, but an estimated one in ten boys in the UK are affected by ADHD. Children with this condition just can't sit still, have volatile moods, get into fights and disrupt their classes. They have a hard time at school and at home, performing badly, getting into trouble and often being shunted from school to school. Furthermore, if left untreated, a hyperactive six-year-old may grow up to become a delinquent teenager.

At a cursory glance, ADHD might look like something to be blamed on poor parenting or schooling, but dig deeper and a plethora of other potential causative factors emerges, including heredity, smoking, alcohol or drug use during the mother's pregnancy, oxygen deprivation at birth, prenatal trauma and environmental pollution. The good news, however, is that, more often than not, children with ADHD have one or more nutritional imbalances, and identifying and correcting these can dramatically improve the children's energy, focus, concentration and behaviour.

### CASE HISTORY *Richard, age eight*

Diagnosed with ADHD, Richard was 'out of control' and his parents were at their wits' end. Richard had also been constipated his entire life, but through biochemical testing at the Brain Bio Centre we found that he was allergic to dairy products and eggs, and was very deficient in magnesium. Dietary analysis revealed that he took in excessive amounts of sugar every day, so we recommended reducing his sugar intake significantly, cutting out dairy and egg products, and supplementing magnesium and omega-3 essential fats. Within three months, his parents reported that Richard had calmed down considerably and had become much more manageable. His constipation had also cleared up completely.

It can be difficult to decide whether your child simply has a great deal of energy or whether they are abnormally active. Use the checklist below to assess your child, scoring two if a symptom is severe, one if it's moderate and zero if it's not present.

## HYPERACTIVITY CHECK

Check whether your child is hyperactive by scoring their characteristics below.

Is your child...

☐ overactive

☐ fidgety

☐ unable to sit still at meals

☐ too talkative

☐ clumsy

☐ unpredictable

☐ unable to respond to discipline

☐ displaying speech problems

☐ unable to listen to a story to the end

☐ hard to get to bed

☐ reckless

☐ impatient

☐ accident-prone

☐ destructive

☐ prone to leave projects unfinished

☐ wears out toys, furniture and so on

☐ uninterested in sticking with games

☐ failing to follow directions

☐ fighting with other children

☐ teasing

☐ 'getting into things'

☐ having temper tantrums

☐ defiant

☐ irritable

☐ unpopular with their peers

☐ lying

☐ wetting the bed

*Score 2 if a symptom is severe, 1 if moderate and 0 if not present. A score of 11 or less is normal. If it's higher, read on to find out more about workable nutritional strategies.*

# Eat to calm down

If your child has ADHD and is eating poorly, the way is clear: you'll need to take a very close look at the amount of refined carbohydrates, harmful trans fats and other problem foods they're consuming, identify what's missing and provide a menu designed to calm them down.

## Show sugar the door

In chapter 2 we saw how vital balanced blood sugar levels are to mental health and advocated a low- or no-sugar diet. A diet high in refined carbohydrates is not good for anyone, but in some children sweet-eating seems to promote hyperactivity and aggression. Essentially, if you feed your child rocket fuel (that is, sugar and caffeine), don't be surprised if their behaviour is out of control. Even so-called 'normal' children can become uncontrollable after a sugarfest, but dietary studies do consistently reveal that hyperactive children eat more sugar than other children[2] and reducing sugar has been found to halve disciplinary actions in young offenders.[3]

Other research has confirmed that the problem is not sugar itself, but the forms it comes in, the absence of a well-balanced diet overall and an abnormal glucose metabolism. A study of 265 hyperactive children found that more than three-quarters of them displayed abnormal glucose tolerance[4] – that is, their bodies were less able to handle their intake of sugar and to maintain balanced blood sugar levels.

In any case, when a child is regularly snacking on refined carbohydrates, sweets, chocolate, fizzy drinks, juices and little or no fibre to slow the glucose absorption, the levels of glucose in their blood will seesaw continually, and trigger wild fluctuations in their levels of activity, concentration, focus and behaviour. These, of course, are also the symptoms of ADHD. The initial calm that sometimes sets in after children eat refined carbohydrates may well be a short-lived normalisation of blood sugar levels from a hypoglycaemic (low blood sugar) state, during which time the brain, including those parts of it that control behaviour, was starved of fuel.

Since children with ADHD seem particularly sensitive to sugar, it's recommended that you remove all forms of refined sugar and any foods that contain it from their diet. This includes processed juices and juice drinks, as they deliver a big shot of sugar very quickly. Replace these with wholefoods and complex carbohydrates, such as brown rice and other whole grains, oats, lentils, beans, quinoa and vegetables, which should be eaten throughout the day – three substantial meals and several snacks will keep blood sugar trickling in slowly and evenly.

To further slow the progress of glucose to their bloodstream, you should ensure that your child's intake of carbohydrates is balanced with protein, so that they eat half as much protein as carbohydrate at every meal and snack. For instance, as we've suggested before, give them a handful of seeds and nuts with a piece of fruit or have chicken or fish with rice for dinner.

## Pump up the essential fats

As we saw in chapter 3, essential fats are crucial for concentration. Omega-3s, in particular, have a clear calming effect on many children with ADHD and, like those with dyslexia, many children with ADHD have visible symptoms of essential fat deficiency, such as excessive thirst, dry skin, eczema and asthma.

It is also interesting that boys, whose requirement for essential fats is much higher than girls', are also much more likely to have ADHD: four out of five sufferers are male. Researchers have theorised that ADHD children may be deficient in essential fats not just because their dietary intake from foods such as seeds and nuts is inadequate (though this is not uncommon), but also because their need is higher, their absorption is poor or they are unable to convert these fats effectively into EPA and DHA, and from DHA into prostaglandins, which are also important for brain function.[5]

Consequently, it's relevant that the conversion of essential fats can be inhibited by most of the foods that cause symptoms in children with ADHD, such as wheat, dairy and foods containing salicylates, compounds which inhibit the conversion and utilisation of essential fats. This conversion is also hindered by deficiencies of the various vitamins and minerals that help the enzymes driving these conversions – vitamin B3 (niacin), B6, C, biotin, zinc and magnesium. Again, zinc deficiency is common in children with ADHD.

Research carried out at Purdue University in the US confirmed that children with ADHD have an inadequate intake of the nutrients required for the conversion of essential fats into prostaglandins, and have lower levels of EPA, DHA and AA than children without ADHD.[6] Supplementation with all these omega-3 essential fats, pre-converted, along with the omega-6 essential fat GLA, reduced ADHD symptoms such as anxiety, attention difficulties and general behaviour problems.[7–8]

Research at Oxford University has proven the value of these essential fats in a trial involving 41 children aged eight to 12 years who had ADHD symptoms and specific learning difficulties. Those children receiving extra essential fats in supplements were behaving and learning better within 12 weeks.[9] The case study below, courtesy of the Hyperactive Children's Support Group, is very relevant here.

### CASE HISTORY *Stephen, age six*

Stephen had a history of hyperactivity, with severely disturbed sleep, and disruptive behaviour at home and at school. Threatened with expulsion from school because of his impossible behaviour, his parents were given two weeks to improve matters. They contacted the Hyperactive Children's Support Group and evening primrose oil was suggested. Since Stephen was too young for capsules and wouldn't take the oil from a spoon, a dose of 1.5g was rubbed into his skin morning and evening. The school was unaware of this, but after five days the teacher tele-phoned the mother to say that never, in 30 years of teaching, had she seen such a dramatic change in a child's behaviour.

After three weeks the evening primrose oil was stopped and one week later the school again complained. The oil was then reintroduced and again its effect clearly showed in Stephen's improved behaviour. It's worth noting that rubbing oil on the skin is not nearly as effective as taking it by mouth, because only a small percentage of it makes it into the body, so Stephen's story is all the more remarkable.

Many children do not eat rich sources of omega-3 essential fats and could benefit from eating more oily fish (wild or organic salmon, sardines, mackerel, fresh tuna) and seeds (flax, hemp, sunflower and pumpkin or their cold-pressed oils). It is also important to replace foods known to hinder the conversion of essential fats to prostaglandins, such as deep-fried foods, while supplementing the nutrients needed for the conversion, such as B vitamins and zinc, as discussed above.

## Sort out the allergies

Of all the avenues so far explored, the link between hyperactivity and food sensitivity is the most established. A study by Dr Joseph Bellanti of Georgetown University in Washington DC found that hyperactive children are seven times more likely to have food aller-gies than other children. According to his research, 56 per cent of hyperactive children aged seven to ten tested positive for food aller-gies, compared to less than 8 per cent of 'normal' children. A sep-arate investigation by the Hyperactive Children's Support Group found that 89 per cent of children with ADHD reacted to food colourings, 72 per cent to flavourings, 60 per cent to MSG, 45 per cent to all synthetic additives, 50 per cent to cow's milk, 60 per cent to chocolate and 40 per cent to oranges.[10] (see chapter 6 for more on food additives).

Other substances often found to induce behavioural changes are wheat, corn, yeast, soya, peanuts and eggs.[11] Symptoms strongly linked to allergy include nasal problems and excessive mucus, ear infections, facial swelling and discolouration around the eyes, tonsillitis, digestive problems, bad breath, eczema, asthma, headaches and bedwetting (see chapter 13 for more on food allergies).

Up to 90 per cent of hyperactive children benefit from eliminating foods that contain artificial colours, flavours and preservatives, processed and manufactured foods, and 'culprit' foods identified by either an exclusion diet or blood test.[12] Some parents have also reported success with the Feingold diet, which removes not only all artificial additives, but also foods that naturally contain salicylates.

Researchers at the University of Sydney in Australia found that three-quarters of 86 children with ADHD reacted adversely to foods with salicylates in them.[13] Salicylates inhibit the conversion and utilisation of essential fats, which we know are often low in hyperactive children. However, the list of foods containing salicylates is very long – it includes prunes, raisins, raspberries, almonds, apricots, canned cherries, blackcurrants, oranges, strawberries, grapes, tomato sauce, plums, cucumbers and Granny Smith apples, many of which are otherwise highly nutritious – so cutting them all out should be considered only as a secondary course of action and must be carefully planned and monitored by a nutritional therapist.

Understanding how a low-salicylate diet helps hyperactive children does offer a useful alternative to such a drastic course of action, though, and so instead of avoiding salicylates it may help to simply increase the supply of essential fats, because that has indeed been shown to work.

## Fix the deficiencies

As we've now seen, research has shown that academic performance improves and behavioural problems diminish significantly when children are given nutritional supplements. Although it is unlikely, on the basis of the studies to date, that ADHD is purely a deficiency disease, most children with this diagnosis *are* deficient in certain key nutrients and do respond very well.

Zinc and magnesium are the most commonly deficient nutrients in people with ADHD. In fact, symptoms of deficiency in these minerals are very similar to the symptoms of ADHD. Low levels of magnesium, for instance, can cause excessive fidgeting, anxious restlessness, insomnia, coordination problems and learning difficulties (if accompanied by a normal IQ).

Polish researchers studying 116 children with ADHD found that 95 per cent of them were deficient in magnesium – a much higher percentage than among healthy children. The team also noted a correlation between levels of magnesium and the severity of symptoms. Supplementing 200mg of magnesium for six months significantly reduced hyperactivity in the children with ADHD, but behaviour in the control group, who received no magnesium, became worse.[14]

Dr Neil Ward of the University of Surrey has come up with a finding that could explain the link between ADHD and such deficiencies. In a study of 530 hyperactive children, Ward found that, compared to children without ADHD, a significantly higher percentage of children with the condition had had several courses of antibiotics in early childhood.[15] Further investigations revealed that children who had had three or more such courses before the age of three tested for significantly lower levels of zinc, calcium, chromium and selenium.[16] This is probably because antibiotics have a disruptive effect on beneficial gut flora and consequently on overall digestive health (see chapter 7 for more on this).

## Kick out the toxic nasties

Looking beyond low levels of essential nutrients, excess anti-nutrients can also induce ADHD symptoms. An example of this is copper, which is found in high levels in some children with ADHD.

Studies have also revealed a link between high aluminium and hyperactivity. Many toxic elements deplete the body of essential nutrients, such as zinc, and may contribute to nutritional deficiencies. A hair mineral analysis to rule out heavy metal intoxication is therefore an important component of an overall nutritional approach (see chapter 6 for more on this).

## The rise of Ritalin

It's a sad fact that many hyperactive children are never evaluated for chemical, allergic or nutritional factors, nor are they treated nutritionally. Instead, when faced with a child who has ADHD, most doctors immediately write a prescription for a habit-forming amphetamine such as Ritalin or Concerta, both of which have many properties similar to those of cocaine. In fact, using brain imaging techniques, Dr Nora Volkow of the Brookhaven National Laboratory in Upton, New York, has shown that Ritalin is actually more potent than cocaine.[17]

Despite these findings, the flood of Ritalin prescriptions shows no sign of abating. Ritalin is now given to up to 20 per cent of children in some American schools, even though researchers assessing its effectiveness have found that it has a negative impact on the behaviour of more children than it helps. By 2004, in the UK, prescriptions for Ritalin and similar drugs had risen to 360,000, at a cost of £12.5 million. That's double the level prescribed in 1999 – and this is only one type of stimulant drug given to children.[18] In the US, more than 8 million children are now on the drug – that's a staggering 10 per cent of all boys between the ages of six and 14.

It's thought that the calming effect of drugs like Ritalin on hyperactive children is because there is not enough of the neurotransmitter noradrenalin in the part of the brain that is supposed to filter out unimportant stimuli. Dr Joan Baizer at the University of Buffalo in upstate New York has shown that while Ritalin was previously thought to have only short-term effects, it actually initiates changes in brain structure and function that remain long after the therapeutic effects have dissipated.[19]

Dr Peter Breggin, a psychiatrist at the International Center for the Study of Psychiatry and Psychology in the US, is an outspoken critic of Ritalin. He says the drug, far from helping children with ADHD, actually damages the brain of the developing child by decreasing blood flow. 'Ritalin does not correct biochemical imbalances – it causes them,' he says, further alleging that negative research results are being suppressed to protect the enormous profits from the drug's sale.

This is not good news when you consider the US Drug Enforcement Agency's list of side-effects from this drug. On top of increased blood pressure, heart rate, respiration and temperature, people taking Ritalin can experience appetite suppression, stomach pains, weight loss, growth retardation, facial tics, muscle twitching, euphoria, nervousness, irritability, agitation, insomnia, psychotic episodes, violent behaviour, paranoid delusions, hallucinations, bizarre behaviours, heart arrhythmias and palpitations, psychological dependence and even death.[20]

Nor does Ritalin work over time. The US National Institutes of Health concluded that there is no evidence of any long-term improvement in scholastic performance on Ritalin.[21] What's more, a child given Ritalin or other stimulant drugs is more likely to become addicted to smoking and abuse other stimulant substances, such as cocaine, later in life. The long and short of it is – don't accept a prescription for these drugs on behalf of your child.[22]

Given the possible effect of Ritalin on noradrenalin deficiency in the brain, it is interesting to note that magnesium plays a key role in promoting the production of noradrenalin. Indeed, sure enough, the vast majority of children are able to stop taking Ritalin after as little as three weeks once they start supplementing 500mg of magnesium daily, but while giving your child up to 200mg of magnesium is perfectly safe, we don't recommend larger amounts unless you are under the guidance of a nutritional therapist. Other nutrients involved in the production of noradrenalin include manganese, iron, copper, zinc, vitamin C and vitamin B6,[23] and many of these nutrients are also involved in the proper metabolism of essential fats.

While there is much you can do yourself, ADHD is a complex condition. As such, it really demands supervision and treatment by a qualified practitioner, who can devise the correct nutritional strategy for your child. Your child's supplement requirements must be individually assessed and they will need to follow an optimally healthy diet. A minimum of three to six months may pass before you see any substantial results, but you may well see a general reduction in hyperactivity and an improvement in your child's powers of concentration very quickly. As your child starts to feel and behave better, the positive feedback they receive from you and their teachers can encourage them to stick to the nutritional programme long term – which is what really produces the best results.

## Summary

To support any child who has hyperactivity or ADHD:

- Follow the guidelines in part 1 regarding nutrients, sugar, essential fats and anti-nutrients.

- Check for potential food allergens, such as wheat, dairy, yeast, soya, chocolate, oranges and eggs.

# Chapter 20

.

# Moving off the autistic spectrum

$F$ew conditions are still as mysterious as autism. The 'autistic spectrum' runs all the way from people unable to speak or deal with others, to high-functioning forms such as Asperger's syndrome. The breadth of this spectrum can be startling. For instance, two of the people who have most profoundly shaped our understanding of nature – Einstein and Newton – are now thought by some to have had Asperger's.

The overlapping conditions mentioned in previous chapters – dyslexia, dyspraxia and ADHD – are often present in autism. For this reason, some people are beginning to feel that this trio of conditions actually belongs in the autistic spectrum, as the highest-functioning forms, but autism is a distinct condition, with specific symptoms. These include difficulties with speech; abnormalities of posture or gesture; problems with understanding the feelings of others; sensory and visual misperceptions, fears and anxieties; and behavioural abnormalities such as compulsive/obsessive behaviour and ritualistic movements. Fits and convulsions are also common in severe autistics.

The US State Department of Developmental Services has found that the incidence of autism more than tripled between 1987 and

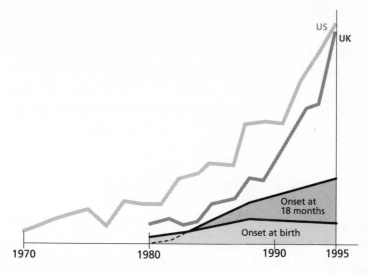

*Autism is on the increase in the US and the UK; The bottom right hand corner illustrates the change in relation to onset of autism*

1999.[1] The figures for the UK range from three to ten times more cases over the last decade or so. While autism used to occur primarily 'from birth' or at least was detected within the first six months, in both the US and UK over the past ten years there has been a dramatic increase in 'late-onset' autism, most frequently diagnosed at age two. According to the UK National Autistic Society, the incidence may now be higher than one in every 100 children.

This strongly suggests that something new is triggering an epidemic. Possible culprits include diet, vaccinations and gastrointestinal problems, which are also very much on the increase in children.

## Andrew, age six

Diagnosed with autism at two and a half, Andrew had frequent ear infections and was a very picky eater, often restricting his diet to just two foods – chicken nuggets and chips. Tests revealed that he had a number of food allergies and was low in magnesium, and an analysis of his diet showed that he was taking in enormous amounts of sugar. Reducing sugar, supplementing magnesium and excluding the foods he was allergic to brought about some significant changes. Within a few weeks, his parents noticed, and others commented, that he seemed much brighter, and more smiley and affectionate. He ceased having ear infections and the range of foods that he would eat broadened considerably.

# Unravelling autism

As with all similar conditions, there is the question of whether autism is 'inherited' or caused by something in a child's diet or environment. Autism is four times as common in boys as girls. Parents and siblings of autistic children are far more likely to suffer from milk or gluten allergy, or have digestive disorders such as irritable bowel syndrome, high cholesterol, night blindness, light sensitivity, thyroid problems or cancer. Not being breast-fed also increases the risk. At first glance, it might seem that autistic children inherit certain imbalances. However, an alternative explanation might be that other family members have the same biochemical imbalances, eat the same food and may be lacking the same nutrients.

Given the overlap with dyslexia, dyspraxia and ADHD, all the factors discussed in previous chapters are also relevant in dealing with autism, so if your child is autistic, you'll need to help them balance blood sugar, check for brain-polluting heavy metals, exclude food additives, identify food allergies, correct digestive problems and possible nutrient deficiencies, and ensure an optimal intake of essential fats. There is growing evidence that these approaches can really make a big difference to children with autism.

## Nutrient deficiencies

We've known since the 1970s that a nutritional approach can help autism, thanks to pioneering research by Dr Bernard Rimland of the Institute for Child Behavior Research in San Diego, California. He showed that vitamin B6, C and magnesium supplements significantly improved symptoms in autistic children. In one of his early studies, back in 1978, 12 out of 16 autistic children improved, then regressed when the vitamins were swapped for placebos.[2]

In the decades following Dr Rimland's study, many researchers have also reported positive results with this approach,[3] but some have failed to confirm positive outcomes with certain nutrients. For example, a French study of 60 autistic children found they improved significantly on a combination of vitamin B6 and magnesium, but not when either nutrient was supplemented alone.[4] This shows how important it is to get the balance of these nutrients right, and the balance is likely to be different for each child.

B6 in particular may help, in part because many children with autism or learning difficulties have a condition in which, for genetic reasons, high levels of a compound called HPL is excreted in the urine, causing a deficiency of zinc and vitamin B6. All children on the autistic spectrum should be screened for urinary HPL. This involves a simple urine test (see Resources) and supplementing with appropriate levels of B6 and zinc, which have brought about remarkable improvements.

## A lack of the right fats

Deficiencies in essential fats are also common in people with autism.[5] Research by Dr Gordon Bell at Stirling University has shown that some autistic children have an enzyme defect that removes essential fats from brain cell membranes more quickly than it should. This means that an autistic child is likely to need a higher intake of essential fats than the average and it has been found that supplementing EPA, which can slow the activity of the defective enzyme, has improved the behaviour, mood, imagination, spontaneous speech, sleep patterns and focus of autistic children.[6–7]

## The link with vitamin A

Paediatrician Mary Megson from Richmond, Virginia, believes that many autistic children are lacking in vitamin A, too. As we've seen, vitamin A, otherwise known as retinol, is essential for vision and it's also vital for building healthy cells in the gut and brain. There's no doubt that something funny is going on in the digestive tracts of autistic children, but how does vitamin A fit into the puzzle?

The best sources of vitamin A are breast milk, organic meats, milk fat, fish and cod liver oil, none of which are prevalent in our diets. Instead, we have formula milk, fortified food and multivitamins, many of which contain altered forms of retinol such as retinyl palmitate, which doesn't work as well as the fish or animal-derived retinol. Megson began speculating what might happen if these children weren't getting enough natural vitamin A.[8]

She realised that not only would this affect the integrity of the digestive tract, potentially leading to allergies, but it would also affect the development of their brains and disturb their vision. Brain differences and visual defects have both been detected in autistic children, and the visual defects, Megson deduced, were an important clue, because lack of vitamin A would mean poor black and white vision, a symptom often seen in the relatives of autistic children.

If you can't see black and white, you can't see shadows and you lose the ability to perceive three-dimensionality. This in turn leaves you less able to make sense of people's expressions, which could explain why some autistic children tend not to look straight at you. Instead, they look at you sideways, which was long thought to be a sign of poor socialisation, but may in fact be the best way for them to see people's expressions, because there are more black and white light receptors at the edge of the visual field than in the middle!

Of course, the proof is in the pudding and Megson has reported rapid and dramatic improvements in autism simply by giving cod liver oil containing natural, unadulterated vitamin A. Often she has seen results within a week of children starting to take the oil.[9] We recommended cod liver oil supplementation for a seven-year-old with Asperger's. As his mother said, 'In the two weeks since following your advice there has been a significant improvement in his eye contact.' Although you need to be careful about the overall amounts of this fat-soluble vitamin your child takes, vitamin A could be an avenue worth pursuing.

Nutrient deficiencies are often made worse by the extremely self-restricted diets that are one of the hallmarks of classic autism. Refusal to eat foods that are not separate on the plate, only eating dry foods or foods of a certain colour, or oral hypersensitivity often make improving the diet of an autistic child extremely challenging. In part 4 we'll give you lots of advice on how to make the changes at a very gradual rate, even in difficult circumstances. The good news, though, is that once a small amount of progress is made, children will often become much more open to trying new foods.

## Allergies – undesirables on board

In addition to these likely deficiencies, the most significant contributing factor in autism appears to be undesirable foods and chemicals that often reach the brain via the bloodstream because of faulty digestion and absorption. Much of the impetus for recognising the importance of dietary intervention has come from parents who've noticed vast improvements in their children after changing their diets. As we've seen elsewhere in this book, certain foods and substances appear to adversely influence a large number of children. These include:

- Wheat and other grains, which contain the protein gluten

- Milk and other dairy products, which contain the protein casein

- Citrus fruits

- Chocolate

- Artificial food colourings

- Paracetamol

- Salicylates

The strongest direct evidence of foods linked to autism involves wheat and dairy, and the specific proteins they contain – namely, gluten and casein. These are difficult to digest and, especially if introduced too early in life, may result in an allergy. Fragments of these proteins, called peptides, can have a big impact in the brain. In fact, they can act directly on the brain by mimicking the body's own natural chemicals or they can disable the enzymes that would otherwise break down these naturally occurring compounds. In either case, the consequence is an increase in chemical activity in the brain, leading to many of the symptoms we describe as autism. Researchers at the Autism Research Unit at Sunderland University have found increased levels of these peptides in the blood and urine of children with autism.[10]

## Gut feelings

To understand how these common foods can be so harmful to sensitive individuals, we need to look at how they get into the body via the gut. As we saw above, peptides, which are sometimes known as exorphins, are derived from incompletely digested proteins, particularly food containing gluten and casein. One of these, which is called IAG and is derived from gluten in wheat, has been detected in 80 per cent of autistic patients.[11] The first problem is therefore the poor digestion of proteins. A lack of sufficient zinc and vitamin B6 could contribute to this, as both are essential for proper stomach acid production and protein digestion, yet autistic children with urinary HPL are often deficient in them, as we saw above.

Whatever the case, how do partially digested protein fragments enter the bloodstream? Vitamin A deficiency is certainly one culprit, but there may be others. Many parents of autistic children report that their child received repeated or prolonged courses of antibiotic drugs for ear or other infections during their first year, before the diagnosis of autism. In chapter 7, we saw how broad-spectrum antibiotics kill good as well as bad bacteria in the gut, weakening the intestinal membranes. This can lead to what is known as leaky gut syndrome, in which large molecules that shouldn't be absorbed through the gut membrane do get through.[12] One kind of these large molecules could be exorphin peptides.

When Dr Andrew Wakefield of London's Royal Free Hospital studied 60 autistic children with gastrointestinal symptoms, he found many more intestinal lesions in them than in non-autistic children with similar digestive problems. In fact, over 90 per cent of the autistic children had chronically inflamed guts as a result of infection.[13] So if your child has autism, restoring their gut to good health is vital. You can start simply, by supplementing digestive enzymes and giving probiotics to restore the balance of gut bacteria. Both measures help heal the digestive tract and promote normal absorption, and have produced positive results in autistic children.[14] Probiotics may also help your child digest exorphins before they can be absorbed.[15]

The amino acid L-glutamine is useful for restoring the integrity of the digestive tract, too. Unfortunately, though, some autistic children cannot process it within their bodies, leading to excess levels of ammonia, so if you wish to try glutamine, do so under the expert guidance of a suitably qualified nutritional therapist.

## Cutting out wheat and dairy

Adding supplements to your child's diet is important, but so is removing any suspect food. There are many anecdotal reports of dramatic improvements in children with autism from parents who removed casein (milk protein) and gluten (the protein in wheat, barley, rye and oats) from their diet.[16] It can take some time for harmful peptides to leave the blood and brain, however, so results can be slow to emerge.

Dr Robert Cade, professor of medicine and physiology at the University of Florida, has observed that as levels of peptides in the blood decrease, the symptoms of autism also decrease. 'If [levels of peptides] can be reduced to normal range,' he says, 'we typically see dramatic improvements.' However, to accomplish this you need to help your child adhere rigidly to a strict gluten/casein-free diet.[17]

If you decide to take this route with your child, you'll need to adopt a go-slow approach. We recommend a gradual withdrawal of foods, waiting three weeks after the removal of dairy foods (casein) before removing wheat, rye, barley and oats (gluten) from the diet. Initially, your child may go through 'withdrawal' and their symptoms may get worse for a while. If this is extreme, you will need to slow down on the removal process. On the plus side, though, their openness to trying new food should improve rapidly once these allergenic foods are reduced or removed.

Keep a food diary and note your child's behaviours and symptoms alongside all the foods they're eating. This can help to identify

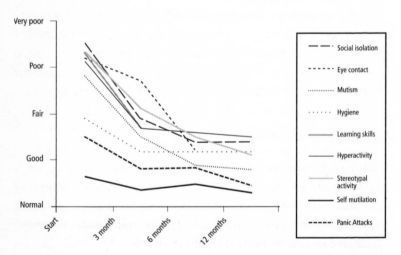

*Symptom improvement in 70 autistic children while on a gluten/casein-free diet over 12 months*

which of the usual suspects they are sensitive to – citrus fruits, chocolate, artificial food colourings, salicylates, eggs, tomatoes, avocados, aubergine, red peppers, soya or corn.[18] Remember, though, that most of the foods in this list contain valuable nutrients as well, so you'll have to ensure that they are replaced rather than just removed. As you'll need to be fully aware of which foods contain gluten and/or casein, this entire process is best done under the guidance of a nutritional therapist (see Resources).

## Tracking down gluten and casein

**Gluten** is found in wheat (and its species and hybrids, spelt, triticale and kamut), oats (different type of gluten to wheat), barley and rye. This means you will need to cut out most bread, biscuits, cakes, pasta, breakfast cereals, bulghur, couscous, pizza, pitta bread, wraps, chapattis, naans, egg noodles, pastry, bagels, crumpets, pot noodles, pies, sausages, ready meals and processed foods. Check ingredient lists carefully and avoid any products containing flour, rusk, malted flake, modified starch or wheat starch. Most alternatives are based on rice or corn and gluten-free breads, pastas, cereals, biscuits, crackers, cakes and bars are now readily available in health food shops and some supermarkets.

**Casein** is found in all dairy products, including cow's milk, butter, cheese, yoghurt, ice cream and milk chocolate. Sometimes goat's or sheep's milk are better tolerated, but you need to remove these from your child's diet, too. Make use of the many soya alternatives now available, including milk, cheese, yoghurt and ice cream. However, soya itself can also be a problem, because some people develop sensitivity to it, so don't rely on it too heavily, and if you suspect your child has developed an intolerance to it use alternatives made from rice and other gluten-free grains, which are now widely available in health food shops.

## Going for detox

Peptides can also harm the autistic child via the liver. This organ is a dedicated cleaner, detoxifying harmful chemicals and breaking down hormones and neurotransmitters. Through a process called sulphation, the liver deactivates excess amounts of many of the neurotransmitters that modulate mood and behaviour, and so keeps the brain in balance. However, 95 per cent of autistic children have low sulphate levels, which may be inadequate for keeping levels of these neurotransmitters in check. Not only that, but reduced sulphation also affects the mucin proteins that line the gastrointestinal tract, making the gut leakier and promoting inflammatory bowel disease. This in turn allows peptides in, where they proceed to reduce sulphate production, so it's a vicious circle.

The enzyme sulphite oxidase also plays a role in sulphate production and levels of it are often low in autistic children. Sulphite oxidase is dependent on adequate levels of the mineral molybdenum, so supplementing this can be helpful – about 20 per cent of autistic children respond well to it.[19] Also potentially helpful in this context is a highly usable form of sulphur called MSM. For advice on dosage, we recommend you consult a qualified nutritional therapist.

Detoxification of the gut can also be worthwhile. Autistic children often have dysbiosis – the presence of undesirable microorganisms in the gut, whether bacteria, yeasts, fungi or parasites. Treatment with anti-fungal drugs such as Nystatin can get remarkable results, but note that children often get worse before they get better. Other less aggressive anti-fungal agents, including caprylic acid from coconut, charcoal and the yeast saccharomyces boulardi, can be equally effective without triggering such severe reactions.

Rather than doing any of this alone, though, we strongly recommend you work with a nutritional therapist, who can advise you and your child on a suitable plan for detoxification (see Resources).

# The big debate – MMR and autism

Does the MMR vaccine trigger autism? The issue has been hotly debated in the press and among concerned parents across the UK. The official line is that there's no good evidence for any link between autism in children and the MMR. Of course, the last thing the medical profession wants is children not to be vaccinated, since that increases the risk of epidemics, but it's true that Dr Andrew Wakefield's research at the Royal Free Hospital,[20] while important, is only the first hint of a problem and it is probably too early to arrive at any firm conclusions.

It is, however, useful to look at what Wakefield actually said in this context: 'Although MMR cannot by any means be described as a cause of autism, a child genetically predisposed to asthma, eczema, food allergy or intolerance, perhaps with possible disruption of the gut flora or with a fungal overgrowth, deficient in vitamins, minerals and essential fats, may be at risk from MMR. For them MMR could be described as the straw that broke the camel's back, tipping the balance of normal childhood development into a retrogressive state.'[21]

For most children, the MMR vaccine is unlikely to be a problem, but having said this, no one really knows the full consequences of giving a child three immune attacks – mumps, measles and rubella – all at the same time. Getting all three illnesses at once simply doesn't occur in nature, so there's a logical argument for single vaccines if a parent so chooses, especially for children with weakened immune systems. Perhaps for children with nutrient deficiencies, a lack of essential fats, and a susceptibility to food allergies, infections and/or gut problems, these triple vaccines really *are* the last straw.

That said, is there any hard evidence against MMR? Firstly, studies have shown a high incidence of autism in children whose mothers had received live virus vaccines (particularly the MMR or rubella vaccine) immediately before conception or immediately following birth.[22] Secondly, there are two classifications of autism: one where autistic traits are noted from birth and one where symptoms are noted at 18 months plus. The onset of autism at 18 months was uncommon until the mid-1980s, when the MMR vaccine came into wide use. After that, the incidence shot up.[23]

According to Dr Bernard Rimland of the Institute for Child Behavior Research in San Diego, the problem may not be the vaccine itself, but a preservative used, until recently, in multi-dose vials of many childhood vaccines. Thimerosal, a preservative containing high levels of mercury, was used in many vaccines up until 2001. Before this, each vaccine injection exposed the child to levels of toxic mercury in excess of the US federal government's own safety guidelines and a child having all their jabs could have received a total of 187.5mcg of mercury – enough to give them heavy metal poisoning.[24]

Mercury is known to inhibit the enzyme that digests gluten and casein, possibly increasing a child's susceptibility to wheat and milk allergy. Thus this heavy metal in vaccines may have had the knock-on effect of contributing to the food allergies we frequently see in autism.

There's another fact that strengthens the link between autism and MMR, which is that many autistic children have been found to have measles antibodies in their gut. It's a little like having a chronic infection and seems to indicate that the triple vaccine makes measles persist. One of the most important allies the body has to fight off this virus is vitamin A and Dr Megson's research (see page 206) indicates that many autistic children lack this key nutrient.

So, although it is too early to say conclusively yea or nay, it is entirely possible that late-onset autism may be triggered by multiple vaccinations, allergies, toxic overload or nutritional deficiencies – and especially combinations of any of these that send a child's gut and brain into distress.

## To vaccinate or not?

The subject of childhood vaccination is an entire book on its own, so we recommend you read *The Truth About Vaccines* by Dr Richard

Halvorsen (see Recommended reading). Dr Halvorsen, a British GP, has researched this subject thoroughly and presents a balanced and scientific view.

## A natural way with autism

It can be hard work, but the optimum nutrition approach to helping your autistic child is much more effective than the available drugs – and has no negative side-effects. It involves healing the digestive tract, avoiding sources of casein and gluten plus any other identified allergens, eating healthy foods, and supplementing nutrients that help support digestion, absorption, liver detoxification, the immune system and the brain.

As for drugs such as Ritalin, these are in any case generally not recommended for 'classic' autism, except when it is accompanied by ADHD. In one survey of 8,700 parents, asked to rate the effectiveness of drugs and other interventions, it was found that Ritalin was the most commonly prescribed, but only 26 per cent reported any improvement in their child, while 46 per cent said their child deteriorated on it. The most efficient drug in this survey, the antifungal Nystatin, was still found to help only 49 per cent of children taking it.[25]

## Fits, convulsions and epilepsy

Profoundly autistic children may be prone to epilepsy. Although it's less common, people on the 'broader' autistic spectrum – including ADHD, dyslexia and dyspraxia – may also have fits or convulsions. Lasting for seconds or minutes, convulsions are thought to be the result of a temporary upset in the brain's chemistry, causing neurons to fire off faster than usual and in bursts.

Neurological problems such as a brain injury, a stroke, an infection and, less frequently, a tumour can all bring on convulsions.

High levels of stress and panic attacks can also trigger them, as can heart disease, especially irregular heartbeats, and blood sugar problems. Whatever the cause, convulsions indicate that the brain is out of balance, so an obvious place to start is to ensure an optimal intake of the brain's best friends – nutrients.

Many researchers have pointed out that people who have epilepsy or convulsions are often deficient in certain nutrients – usually folic acid, the minerals manganese and magnesium, essential fats and vitamin D.

## Nutrients that counter convulsions

**B vitamins** Folic acid is depleted by convulsions, suggesting that it is somehow involved in them,[26] so it is ironic that anti-convulsant drugs such as phenytoin, primidone and phenobarbital further deplete folic acid.

Combining a drug such as phenytoin with folic acid works better than the drug alone. In one study, epileptics were given this drug with either folic acid or a placebo, and after a year only those on folic acid reported substantially fewer fits.[27] However, folic acid could be a double-edged sword. Some studies without control groups suggest that supplementation with this nutrient may actually cause epileptic fits in a minority of people. Several controlled studies, however, have failed to confirm this observation, suggesting that the incidence must be very rare.[28] With the guidance of your doctor, folic acid supplementation is well worth trying, although you can't expect immediate results.

Also worth supplementing is vitamin B6, which in high doses can produce almost immediate results. The first research to identify a role for B6 in the treatment of epilepsy in children took place in Japan in the 1980s. More than half the children with 'infantile spasms' responded very well to B6 supplementation, although the doses used were very high and did cause side-effects in some participants.[29]

In a more recent study at the University of Heidelberg in Germany, 17 children were given high doses of vitamin B6 (300mg/kg/day). Five out of the 17 had immediate relief within two weeks, while after four weeks all the patients were more or less free of seizures. No serious adverse reactions were noted. The side-effects were mainly gastrointestinal symptoms and they were reversed after the dosage was reduced.[30]

**Manganese, magnesium and zinc** The mineral manganese is essential for proper brain function and, to date, four studies have shown a correlation between low levels of it and epilepsy, suggesting that as many as one in three children with epilepsy have low manganese levels.[31–32]

In one study, published in the *Journal of the American Medical Association*, one child found to have half the normal blood manganese levels didn't respond to any medication, but on supplementing manganese had fewer seizures, and improved speech and learning.[33] The late Dr Carl Pfeiffer, one of the pioneers of nutritional medicine, was the first to report the successful treatment of epilepsy with manganese.[34] At the Brain Bio Centre we have frequently found that patients with fits or convulsions are manganese-deficient and have no or fewer fits once supplementation has begun.

Manganese is found mainly in seeds, nuts, grains and tropical fruit, such as bananas and pineapples. (Tea is very rich in it, but we categorically do not recommend children drink tea, as it's a stimulant.)

Magnesium is another mineral well worth checking out if your child is having fits or convulsions. Magnesium is vital for proper nerve and brain function, and, once again, a number of researchers have found low levels in patients with epilepsy and reported fewer fits on supplementation.[35–36] In animals, magnesium injections have also been shown to instantly suppress convulsions.[37]

Supplementing with magnesium is especially helpful for those with 'temporal lobe' epilepsy, where a person has hallucinations of sound or smell, say, before a fit. This is hopeful news for children with this type of epilepsy, as they rarely respond to conventional anti-convulsant drugs.[38] It is also possible that the children of women who are deficient in manganese while pregnant with them are more likely to be born with epilepsy.

Finally, it's also well worth testing for zinc, as children with epilepsy can have lower levels of this mineral[39] and anti-convulsant drugs can deplete it further. There is also data suggesting that having high levels of copper and a lack of zinc may increase the odds of having a seizure[40] – ideally, we need to take in ten times more zinc than copper. Zinc is also a valuable ally for vitamin B6, since it helps convert B6 (pyridoxine) into the active form of the vitamin, called pyridoxal-5-phosphate. It is highly likely that the few children who have had adverse reactions to very high doses of vitamin B6 might not have done so if they had been given B6 together with zinc.

In fact, most adverse reactions to vitamins or minerals arise when they are treated like drugs and given at very high doses without other nutrients, thereby completely ignoring the principle of synergy, whereby nutrients working together amplify each others' action. For this reason, we strongly recommend that if your child is experiencing fits, convulsions or epilepsy, you see a nutritional therapist for a thorough nutritional workout.

This should involve both hair and blood analyses for manganese, magnesium and zinc, as well as folic acid. Levels of magnesium and folic acid are best tested in red blood cells. Depending on the results, a nutritional therapist can work out what combination of these nutrients, often in high doses, are worth trying, together with basic multivitamin supplementation.

An all-round good diet and supplements programme is, in fact, especially important for children with epilepsy, since other nutrients have also been shown to have positive effects on mental health in epileptics. These include vitamin B1,[41] selenium[42] and vitamin E.[43]

**Vitamin D** A deficiency in vitamin D may both contribute to seizures and be worsened by epilepsy medication.[44-45] Vitamin D helps the body to take up calcium, so deficiency in this vitamin can lead to a severe calcium deficiency, one symptom of which is seizures. Several anticonvulsant drugs interfere with the metabolism of vitamin D in the body, which may contribute to or worsen a deficiency. However, there is a paucity of research in this area, with only one pilot study showing that supplementation of vitamin D reduced seizures,[46] and until more is known we advise that you have your child's vitamin D levels tested if they have seizures or are on anticonvulsant medication. The best source of vitamin D is sunshine, which is not widely available in the UK for many months of the year, so if your child has a low level, supplementation will be required. For severe deficiency, higher doses may be required under the supervision of a nutritional therapist or paediatrician.

**Essential fats** One of the hottest areas of research into epilepsy is the effect of essential fat deficiency. So many people are deficient in omega-3s, in fact, that it's highly likely that a significant proportion of people with epilepsy are also deficient; and there is intriguing evidence to show that supplementation can reduce the incidence of convulsions.

In one study, omega-3 and omega-6 essential fats, in a ratio of 1:4, were given to epileptic rats. After three weeks, up to 84 per cent fewer of the rats were having seizures and the seizures that did occur tended to be very brief – there was up to a 97 per cent reduction in their duration. The team of researchers think this result was down to the positive effect of essential fats on stabilising signals between brain cells.[47]

Omega-3s also work in humans. Researchers at the Kalanit Institute for Retarded Child in Israel gave children with epilepsy 3g of omega-3 fats for six months and found a dramatic reduction in both the number and severity of epileptic seizures.[48]

For some years there has been a widely held, but unsupported view, that omega-6 supplementation may increase the risk of seizures. Fortunately, a recent review of the evidence by Professor

Basant Puri of Imperial College, London has found that the opposite may be true. Omega-6 essential fats are not only safe for epileptics but may also reduce seizure activity.[49]

**Amino acids, phospholipids and herbs** Many of the 'brain food' nutrients discussed in part 1, including phosphatidyl choline and essential fats, may also be helpful for children prone to fits. The brain's 'master tuners' – the amino acids SAMe and TMG – are also potential aids (see chapter 18 for more on this). A close relative of these, DMG (di-methyl glycine), produced remarkable results in one 22-year-old man with long-standing learning disabilities, who had been having around 17 seizures a week, despite taking anticonvulsant medication. Within one week of starting 90mg of DMG twice a day, his seizures dropped to just three a week. When the DMG was withdrawn twice, the frequency of his seizures increased dramatically both times.[50]

The amino acid taurine, which helps to calm down the nervous system, may also help. In animals studies, low concentrations of taurine have been found in parts of the brain where seizure activity is highest and supplementing taurine was found to have a potent, selective and long-lasting anticonvulsant effect.[51]

The real star among these amino acids, though, has got to be GABA, the brain's peacemaker, because it acts directly as a neurotransmitter. One possible mechanism for explaining why anticonvulsant drugs work is that they block the activity of the excitatory neurotransmitter, glutamic acid, and thereby promote the inhibitory neurotransmitter, GABA.

However, we would be cautious about supplementing GABA, and possibly large amounts of taurine, except under medical supervision. This is mainly because animal studies have shown that rats prone to petit mal seizures (where they seem 'absent' and stare blankly) sometimes have too much of these amino acids.[52]

Another brain-friendly nutrient, DMAE, while potentially helpful, should also be given with caution. This is because, while DMAE is very helpful for many children with ADHD, a small percentage find it overstimulates, so it should be used with caution in children with manic tendencies or a history of epilepsy, ideally under the guidance of a nutritional therapist.

Vinpocetine, a herbal extract derived from the periwinkle plant (vinca minor), may also help with fits, according to research in Russia.[53] This extract does many useful things in the brain, such as improving the production of cellular energy in neurons, and widening blood vessels so glucose and oxygen get to the brain more easily, and are used more efficiently. As one theory about epileptic fits is that they're caused by fluctuations in glucose or oxygen supplies to the brain, this might explain why vinpocetine works.

So, the message here is that if your child is prone to fits, convulsions or epilepsy and hasn't been checked out by a nutritional therapist, there is plenty of room for hope.

## Summary

If your child has autism, to support them:

- Follow the recommendations at the end of chapters 11 and 19.

- Completely eliminate gluten and dairy from your child's diet and replace them with the now readily available alternatives, while also checking the possibility of other food sensitivities under the guidance of a nutritional practitioner.

- Give your child cod liver oil, vitamin B6, magnesium, zinc, vitamin C, molybdenum and high-strength probiotics (minimum 4 billion microorganisms) daily.

- Ask your nutritional therapist to check your child for urinary HPL and, if they have it, include zinc and vitamin B6 in the above supplement regime.

- When considering the MMR vaccination, if your child has a weak immune system or you suspect nutrient deficiencies,

continues →

low essential fats, susceptibility to food allergies, infections and/or gut problems, consider giving them single vaccines if they are available. Alternatively, address all these issues with a nutritional therapist prior to their receiving the triple vaccine.

If your child has fits, convulsions or epilepsy, to support them:

- Balance your child's blood sugar and check for food allergies.

- Have their vitamin and mineral levels checked. If they are low in folic acid, B6, magnesium, manganese, zinc and vitamin D, supplementation may well help.

- Make sure they are getting enough essential fats, from seeds, fish and their oils.

- Other brain-friendly nutrients and herbs, including amino acids, phosphatidyl choline, DMAE, taurine and vinpocetine may help, but they are best taken under professional guidance.

# PART 4

·

# FOOD FOR THOUGHT

Now that you know what optimum nutrition for your child really means, how do you put this into action? In this part we'll show you what to do to feed your child properly, from infancy to teenage years. You'll find masses of tips and practical ways to keep your child's diet on track, and help choosing the right supplements.

# Chapter 21

·

# Getting off to a good start

Ideally, optimum nutrition for your child starts with you. If you're optimally nourished before you even conceive, and all the way through pregnancy and breast-feeding, you're giving your child a brilliant head start in life.

Breast milk is, of course, your child's optimum food for robust physical and mental health during those crucial first few months. Developing good food habits starts with the weaning process, when your two main objectives need to be keeping your child from developing food allergies and ensuring they develop a taste for a wide range of healthy foods.

## The smart way to feed your baby

As a way of nourishing your baby, breast-feeding is better by design. Breast-fed babies are not only healthier all round, less prone to allergies in later life,[1] with a lower risk of infections and auto-immune disease, they are also smarter! A recent series of worldwide studies indicates that breast-fed babies have an IQ six to ten points higher than that of formula-fed babies.[2]

One reason for this is probably the high levels of the omega-3 fat DHA that's found naturally in breast milk. As we've seen, DHA is vital for brain development and the longer a baby is breast-fed, the higher the intelligence they can expect to have as young adults.[3] Another reason for their higher intelligence is likely to be that the fat-soluble vitamins in breast milk are more easily absorbed.

In a Brazilian study, only one in 176 breast-fed babies had lower than adequate levels of vitamin E, compared to more than half in a cow's milk formula-fed group.[4] Another study has shown that breast milk is higher in vitamin D than formula milk – and not just any vitamin D, but a particular kind which has been found to be two and a half times more effective at preventing rickets, the deficiency disease in which bones don't develop properly, which, amazingly, is on the increase in Britain.[5] There are also more brain-boosting minerals in breast milk than in most formulas.[6]

Breast-feeding also helps to establish healthy gut bacteria. A type of beneficial gut bacteria called bifidobacteria, present in breast but not formula milk, prevents harmful bacteria from invading your baby's gut. This is an important service, as it not only protects against colic, eczema and asthma, but crucially, as we saw in chapter 13, also helps to prevent food allergies.

Breast-fed babies are also less likely to be obese. A study of 32,000 Scottish three- to four-year-olds found that those breast-fed for six to eight weeks after birth were 30 per cent less likely to be obese than bottle-fed children.[7]

Breast-feeding has benefits for the mother too, with a quicker and easier return to your pre-pregnancy weight, because you're using 500 extra calories a day to breast-feed. You're also at lower risk of breast and ovarian cancer later in life if you breast-feed. What's more, breast milk is more convenient than formula feeding. It's on tap, always at the right temperature, requires no bottles or mixing, and, of course, it's cheaper, too. For more information on healthy nutrition during pregnancy, breast-feeding, and the best alternatives to breast milk, read *Optimum Nutrition Before, During and After Pregnancy* by Patrick Holford and Susannah Lawson (see Recommended reading).

# Keeping your child allergy-free

As with so much else, prevention is better than cure, and preventing an allergy from developing in your child is much easier and better than trying to 'cure' it later. There are two important points here. One is the choice and timing of first foods, the other the health of your baby's digestive system.

## When to wean

Don't start weaning your child on to food earlier than you need to – start at around six months. It's preferable to breast-feed your baby exclusively up to this point. If they are failing to thrive on breast milk alone, visit your paediatrician and a nutritional therapist for advice before deciding to add other foods to their diet. A lack of solid foods or formula milk may not be the problem and adding these to their diet may make things worse if poor digestion is an issue.

The right time to wean will vary from baby to baby, so fortunately there are several signs of readiness to look for. Your baby may be ready for solid foods if they start to show an interest in what you're eating and seem to want to try some. By this time, they should also be able to sit up, pick up food and put it in their mouth. They will also have lost the 'tongue-thrusting reflex' that causes them to automatically push solids out of their mouth. This natural reflex protects babies from choking when they are too young for solids. For some babies, there may be a connection between how they 'mouth' their toys and how ready they are for solid foods. Up to the age of six months, babies tend to place toys and other objects in their mouths, but 'mouth' them in a random fashion. However, after six months of age, they tend to display a much greater interest in actually discovering the texture and shape of an object with their mouths, tongues and lips. Watch your baby closely for this type of behaviour when they place objects in their mouth – it's another clue that they're ready to add solid food to their diet.

Appearing hungrier is not a reliable sign that your baby is ready for solid food as babies sometimes show appetite spurts and may simply need more breast milk or formula. Most babies start to cut their teeth at around six months, which helps with biting and chewing food. Some babies do get their first teeth earlier than this and a baby who is unsettled and putting his fists in his mouth a lot may be teething rather than hungry. Weaning early will not help your baby sleep through the night. In fact, the opposite may be true if they develop food allergies.

## Pureed vs solid

Learning to chew – either with teeth or gums – is an important part of your baby's development, because it strengthens the jaw muscles, helps with the development of speech, helps to promote healthy teeth and enables your baby to enjoy finger foods and other items that the rest of the family are eating. Pureed foods can be used for younger babies, but shouldn't be continued longer than is necessary.

If you're struggling to get your baby to take lumpy foods – and assuming they are showing all the right signs of readiness – try feeding your baby on your lap. They may be reassured by the closeness and more likely to experiment with their food. They may even accept a little lumpy, but suitable, food from your plate. Ensure that mealtimes are fun. Try singing to your baby and smile often. Praise them lavishly for any progress they make. Always eat with your baby – babies love to mimic others and watching you may be just the incentive yours needs. Offer your baby plenty of finger foods if they're developmentally ready. Many babies won't take lumpy foods from a spoon, but will chew quite happily when feeding themselves! Encourage your baby to explore toys with their mouth. This helps to develop the tongue movement, which is needed to gather and chew particles of food. Hungry babies are more easily frustrated with the new feeding experience, so often a small milk feed to take the edge of their appetite before offering the solid food works best. Most important of all, don't panic! Anxiety on your part won't help.

## First foods

Vegetables make good first foods. Cooked carrot, potato, parsnip, turnip and sweet potato can be chopped, sieved or mashed, the smoothness depending on your baby's age. If you start weaning earlier than six months, the food will need to be pureed, but for babies of around six months or more food can simply be mashed with a fork. Indeed, some babies immediately cope with soft finger foods such as cooked carrots or a piece of pear. For a younger baby you can add expressed breast milk, formula or the water the vegetables were cooked in. Gluten-free grains such as rice and quinoa are also suitable. They can be boiled or ground and, again, mixed with a little breast milk, formula or boiled water. Never add salt to a baby's food, either at the cooking stage or afterwards.

Home-made foods are nutritionally superior to pre-prepared or 'baby foods' that come in jars. They're fresh, nutritious, you know exactly what's in them and they haven't been through any preservation processes. They are also considerably cheaper and, because they can contain a single ingredient, it's easier to keep track of how your baby takes to each new food you introduce.

### WHAT TO INTRODUCE WHEN WEANING

#### From six months

- Vegetables *except* tomatoes, potatoes, peppers and aubergines (members of the 'deadly nightshade' family)
- Fruits *except* citrus
- Pulses and beans
- Rice, quinoa, millet and buckwheat
- Fish (preferably organic, wild or deep sea)

**From nine months**
- Meat and poultry (preferably organic)
- Oats, corn, barley and rye
- Live yoghurt
- Tomatoes, potatoes, peppers and aubergines
- Eggs
- Soya (tofu or soya milk)

**From 12 months**
- Citrus fruits
- Wheat
- Dairy products
- Nuts and seeds

To begin with, introduce only one food each day, make a note of it in your weaning diary and watch for any possible reaction. This could be anything from a skin rash or eczema, excessive sleepiness, a runny nose, an ear infection, dark circles under the eyes, excessive thirst, over-activity, wheezing, colic, diarrhoea or stool changes (consistency, colour and smell). If you notice anything amiss, stop giving that food and then introduce another once the reaction has died down. You can double-check your observations by reintroducing these foods a few months later. By that time your baby's digestive system will have matured, so they should no longer react to that food. If your baby still shows a strong reaction to this particular food, it would be sensible to see your paediatrician and a nutritional therapist for advice on supporting your baby's digestive system.

Once your baby is eating a mixture of foods that cause no reaction, it's then important to vary their diet as much as possible, especially with common allergenic culprits such as wheat, dairy, soya and citrus fruits. Eating the same thing over and over again can overtax the system and induce an allergy, plus a varied diet will also boost your child's desire for a wider range of foods, which will in turn ensure they're getting a broader range of nutrients.

## Drinks

Breast milk (or formula) will be the main source of liquid for the first year, but water can be offered in a beaker or cup with meals. This is especially important if you are formula feeding, as if babies are thirsty they may take more formula milk than they need. Don't give your baby fruit juice to drink for at least their first year, even if it's diluted. It can damage their teeth, as their tooth enamel is not as strong as an adult's.

## Digestive health

Food allergies are intimately linked to poor digestive health – one seems to exacerbate the other – but keeping your baby's gut healthy is vital for many other reasons, too. For instance, gut and brain are closely connected via the nervous system; so closely that the gut can actually be thought of as a second brain. Called the enteric nervous system, the network of neurons, neurotransmitters and proteins lining the gut is in constant communication with your child's central nervous system, up in their brain and spinal cord, so keeping their gut healthy is essential for optimising their brain development.

Unfortunately, many babies these days seem to have their first dose of antibiotics within days or weeks of birth, resulting in gastric upsets and more. As we've seen, antibiotics wipe out the beneficial gut flora in the digestive tract, causing an imbalance that can lead to food allergies, digestive problems and lower levels of essential minerals.

Antibiotics are often given to babies for ear, nose and throat infections, which may themselves be caused by food allergies, particularly if they are recurrent, so it is well worth getting to the root of the problem and resolving food allergies. According to a study published in the *Journal of the American Medical Association*, antibiotics given for ear infections in children triples the chance of a repeat infection![8]

While breast milk contains beneficial gut flora that will recolonise your baby's gut following antibiotics, formula milk typically doesn't. If it's essential for your baby to take antibiotics, make sure you follow them with an age-appropriate probiotic supplement that will supply the right strains of gut flora (see Products and supplements directory).

## Establishing healthy eating

Once your child is successfully on to solids, the next 18 months are absolutely crucial to establishing healthy eating. The emphasis should be on vitamin- and mineral-rich vegetables and fruit, and good quality protein. Choose organic if you can, so you are not polluting your baby with residues from artificial fertilisers, herbicides or pesticides.

Many parents make the mistake of weaning their child on to a lot of fruit and 'baby cereals', both of which are very sweet. If you do this, you may find your child rejecting vegetables, so really prioritise vegetables over fruit until your baby is happily eating a variety of veg. The less sweet food and drink your baby has, the less they will desire it. Also, remember that while you're feeding broccoli to your baby, they will be watching your facial expression, so look like you enjoy eating it, too! It's very easy to unconsciously let your face screw up into a grimace while cooing 'Mmmm yummm' to your baby. They won't be fooled if your *face* is saying 'Ooh yuck!'

Make sure, too, that you give your baby foods that have a range of different colours. Dr Gillian Harris, a clinical psychologist at Birmingham University in the UK, has studied the impact of first foods on a child's food preferences later on. She found that babies weaned on rusks, baby food, processed foods and milk are more likely to go on to prefer 'beige carbohydrates' such as crisps, white bread and chips, rather than eating their greens. Babies exposed to fruit, vegetables and a range of other 'non-beige' foods will, by contrast, show a greater preference for many-hued, nutrient-laden foods later on.

Dr Harris puts this down to an ancient survival mechanism. She believes that children build up a 'visual prototype' of favoured foods. This model meshes with evolutionary theory, which suggests that our tastes and preferences were shaped to help us survive.

We are born with a love of sweet tastes, associated with ripe fruit and breast milk, and a dislike of bitter tastes, linked for obvious survival reasons with alkaloid toxins in plants. We can learn to change these tastes depending on what our parents give us to eat, but at the age of around 18 months, when a Stone Age toddler would have been able to wander around and select their own food for the first time, the visual prototype mechanism is turned on to prevent them from wanting to eat unfamiliar and potentially poisonous foods. Many parents report that their child was a 'good eater' until the age of two or three and that suddenly they started refusing everything until their diet narrowed to a handful of foods. To prevent this from happening it's crucial at this point to keep the variety in their diet; it's much more difficult to broaden their diet later than it is to keep the variety up from the start.

## Does my child need to drink milk?

For as long as you breast-feed, you don't need to supplement your baby's diet with cow's milk. However, once you stop, you will need to ensure they get a good source of calcium. Milk has been marketed for decades as the perfect calcium-rich food, especially for young children, but the key word here is 'marketed'.

Early humans drank no milk after weaning, yet they still managed to develop strong bones and teeth. There is no evidence that once they ceased to be nomadic hunter-gathers and began to cultivate the land, eating grains and keeping animals for meat and milk, their bones got stronger. In fact, the opposite seems to be true and we appear to have shrunk in height by about 15cm! This, however, is thought to be due to difficulties in dealing with grain, rather than any problem with milk.[9]

We need to remember that milk is a specialised food full of hormones geared for calves, rather than us, and, as we've seen, milk protein or casein causes digestive problems in many people. Meanwhile, if it is so essential, where do the Chinese, for instance, whose consumption of milk is exceedingly low, get their calcium from? The answer is from vegetables, nuts, seeds and soya products, so while it's widely consumed by our society, milk doesn't seem to stand up as an essential for good health. Also, as many people develop allergies to it, it's not a good idea for your child to become too reliant on milk, as long as you make sure their diet is rich in other sources of calcium. See the table opposite for the best calcium-rich foods, which are important inclusions in your child's diet if they're avoiding dairy products.

If you decide you do want to give your child milk, reduce its allergic potential by rotating cow's milk with goat's and sheep's milk, plus soya, rice and oat milks. Visit your local health food shop to find a full selection. We ourselves buy a variety and switch between them, using up one carton before starting on a different type of milk.

Yoghurt is often better tolerated than milk, as the live bacteria that make it predigest a lot of the problematic milk sugars and proteins. Live yoghurt, where this bacteria remains intact, can be particularly helpful in promoting a healthy digestive system and the calcium in yoghurt is easier to absorb than that in milk. Goat's and sheep's yoghurt is also easy to find these days, allowing you more variety.

## CALCIUM IN FOODS – THE RICHEST SOURCES

| per 100g/100ml | Calcium content (mg) |
| --- | --- |
| Cheddar cheese | 720 |
| Tahini (sesame seed paste) | 680 |
| Sesame seeds | 670 |
| Sardines canned in oil | 550 |
| Almonds | 240 |
| Spring greens | 210 |
| Watercress | 170 |
| Brazil nuts | 170 |
| Kale | 150 |
| Tofu (enriched with calcium) | 150 |
| Blackstrap molasses (per tablespoon) | 150 |
| Whole milk | 115 |

# Summary

To get your child off to the best start in life:

- Breast-feed your baby exclusively for six months, then wean them following the guidelines in this chapter. Continue feeding some breast milk for a full 12 months. If you're formula feeding, seek advice from a qualified nutritional therapist to ensure your baby isn't missing out on any nutrients.

- During weaning, introduce plenty of colourful vegetables rather than bland, sweet fruit or cereal mixes, and as you demonstrate eating it to your baby, look like you're enjoying it, too!

- If your baby is given antibiotics, follow them with age-appropriate probiotics to replenish the beneficial gut flora. Seek advice from a nutritional therapist.

# Chapter 22

·

# The pot of gold

By the age of 18 months to two years, your child will be eating pretty much the same foods as the rest of the family, providing, of course, that the rest of the family isn't eating highly salted or spicy food! In this chapter we outline in detail the ideal diet for all children. Remember this is the ideal diet and may be only something to aspire to, but at least you know what you're aiming for.

## Breakfast

The ideal breakfast consists of low GL carbohydrates combined with some protein, nuts and/or seeds for the essential fats and minerals, and fruit to provide those all important antioxidants.

There are three main categories of breakfast: cereal, something on toast or a liquid breakfast.

### Cereal

Obviously, the sugar-laden children's favourites such as Frosties, Crunchy Nut cornflakes and Coco Pops are off the menu entirely.

They are nutritionally poor, being high GL, high in refined sugar and carbs, and very sweet to taste, so they promote a sweet tooth. Eating these, your child will probably be hyped up, but will only feel full briefly before their blood sugar plummets and they're craving their next sugar hit.

Next on the list to discard are the less sugar-laden, but equally refined cereals. Here we're talking about puffed rice and cornflakes and the like. The sugar is less obvious, but these products still have a very high GL. In fact, we describe puffed rice to our young charges as sugar-coated air – the high GL crispy rice carbs being equivalent to sugar – and as such they're not a good choice for the most important meal of the day. Weetabix and Bran Flakes are a medium GL choice, but the heavy wheat bran content plays havoc with many a digestive tract. Bran flakes with added dried fruit, such as Fruit and Fibre, are also heavy on the wheat bran and the GL is a bit higher. Finally, beware of the 'crunchy cluster' cereals. Although the packet may call it something different, the clusters are held together by sticky stuff called sugar.

Oats undoubtedly make the best cereal-type breakfast. They're low GL, less allergenic (80 per cent of coeliacs can tolerate oats) and unrefined so retain their nutrients. Even some children on a gluten-free diet who are not coeliac can eat oats, because oats don't contain the more problematic type of gluten called gliadin. Instead, they contain a version called avenin, which seems to be better tolerated.

Raw oats are the base of a good muesli. Since most 'shop-bought' mueslis are heavy on the dried fruit, the best muesli is a home-made one. Simply buy a bag of oats, a couple of bags of nuts and a couple of bags of seeds. For variety, use some of the other whole grains available from health food shops, such as buckwheat, quinoa or rye flakes. Quinoa is particularly good because its high protein content makes it especially low GL and it's a good source of the essential amino acids. Mix it up in your plastic muesli container and it's done. You could add a small amount of dried fruit to the mix, but it's even better to serve with plenty of fresh fruit – lower GL, more of those wonderful antioxidants and a lovely natural sweetness. Other sweeteners might include a little apple juice or xylitol if absolutely necessary. Softening the oats by adding a little water (cold or hot) means you need less milk or yoghurt. We recommend using a variety of milks and yoghurts – cow's, sheep's, goat's, soya, quinoa, oat and rice.

Cooked oats, aka porridge, are especially good in winter and they've certainly experienced a resurgence in popularity in recent years. Again, you can also use other flaked grains such as buckwheat, quinoa or rye, or a mix, for variety. Gone are the days of boring old porridge – welcome in the era of super porridge! There's a whole range of yummy foods to add. Fresh fruit gives porridge a real boost. Our favourites are freshly grated apple or fresh (or frozen) raspberries. Grated apple is best added midway through cooking the porridge and works very well with some ground cinnamon. Raspberries are usually better added towards the end if you want to retain their shape or towards the beginning if your kids like the idea of a bowl of red porridge – either way it's delicious. Any fruit will do, so be adventurous.

Creamed coconut or coconut milk added during cooking makes for a lovely creamy coconutty porridge. Coconut creams and milks are high in saturated fat, but remember that children do need some saturated fat in their diet and coconut is a good source. Creamed coconut is particularly convenient because it comes in a solid block, which you can keep in the fridge, using a knob as needed. Don't stop there, though. Try whizzing up some almonds or other nuts and seeds in the grinder for a delicious nutty flavour. Nuts and seeds should be added after the porridge has been removed from the heat, so the wonderful essential fats are not damaged by the cooking. Remember, if you rinse out the saucepan immediately or at least fill it with water it will be very easy to clean later if you're rushing off to do the school run.

You might be tempted to try some of the 'quick oats' or 'microwave oats' available from the supermarket, but they are a poor alternative for several reasons. They often have added sugar and therefore a higher GL, the oats are a much finer ground, which also contributes to a higher GL, and microwaving food is something we prefer to avoid as much as possible.

## Something on toast

The 'something' in the 'something on toast' breakfast needs to be a protein to complement the carbohydrate in the bread and, of course, the toast needs to be a nutritious wholegrain bread. To really complete it, a piece of fruit, and some nuts and seeds, would be ideal, but these can be eaten later in the day or perhaps in the car on the way to school.

What sort of toast? The best bread tends to be the heaviest, darkest, grainiest and least spongy. For kids who can tolerate gluten, a good wheat or rye loaf is usually easy to source. Check the labels and don't choose a bread where the ingredient list looks like it belongs in a chemical factory. When choosing gluten-free breads, you'll find the best selection in health food shops and the better supermarkets. Some of the gluten-free breads, especially those that most closely resemble a white loaf, are loaded with sugar and all sorts of weird-sounding ingredients. Look for the heavy, grainy breads and check the ingredient list. These breads don't really work for sandwiches, but are ideal for toast, although they can take some getting used to. If your kids are off yeast, then sourdough or soda bread are good options. Sourdough rises with the aid of yeast and bacteria that surround us in the air, rather than added baker's yeast, so it's suitable for everyone except those with a very severe yeast allergy. Soda bread is made using baking soda, although it usually contains some dairy produce, too.

If you can't find a bread that your gluten-free, yeast-free child will eat, you need to look to other sources of carbohydrates for breakfast. Potatoes or other starchy vegetables, cold from last night's roast or gently heated, work well with eggs. The middle-eastern falafel, made from chickpeas, can be eaten cold or grilled in a few minutes. Brown rice kedgeree is quick and easy, especially if you have rice left over from the previous evening, or reheat some leftover pasta and mix in some sauce, although you'll need to add some protein to complete the breakfast, of course (see below).

On the whole, butter is better than margarine, even one that makes fantastic health claims. If your child is allergic to dairy, then choose a margarine that's free from trans fats and where the ingredient list includes only recognisable food ingredients. Lactose intolerance is an inability to digest milk sugars (lactose) and dairy allergy is a reaction to milk protein (casein), so those with a mild dairy allergy may be fine with butter, since it is almost pure fat.

For the topping choose a good protein source. This could be an egg, baked beans, unsweetened nut butter (such as peanut butter or the more exotic almond, cashew or hazelnut butter), pumpkin seed butter, hummus or fish (sardines, mackerel, kippers or smoked salmon with a squeeze of lemon juice). Avocado is also brilliant on toast with a slice of tomato – it's not a high protein food but it is high in nutritious fats, so like the protein foods, it lowers the GL of the breakfast. If none of these appeal, good quality sausages, gently grilled bacon or home-made meatballs are great sources of protein, if a little high in saturated fat.

Jam, marmalade, honey, syrup, Nutella or Marmite are not good toast toppings, because they don't have the sustaining power of the proteins (or fat in the case of avocado). Of course, they can be eaten from time to time, especially at the end of a big weekend breakfast, but they just shouldn't be standard breakfast fare.

If your child likes a variety of finger foods to nibble, give them toast soldiers, chopped pieces of boiled egg, a few pieces of fruit and some nuts arranged on a plate.

## The liquid breakfast

A super-smoothie is the best breakfast for those who can't face eating food in the morning. It needs to be substantial enough to keep them going, so while a fresh fruit and/or vegetable juice is super nutritious, its not enough on its own. As with the other breakfast options, the criteria is a low GL and nutrient-rich mix. Fruit is a good source of carbs – go easy on the bananas – and can be combined with oat or quinoa flakes, seeds and nuts, and a dairy or non-dairy milk or yoghurt.

# Lunch

In our ideal world, this meal would consist of about one quarter protein, one quarter carbohydrate and half non-starchy vegetables. In other words, a ratio of 1:1:2.

## School meals

If your child is eating at nursery or school, you'll need to find out what's on offer. Most school caterers will have a three-week rotating menu and will be able to provide you with a copy. Unfortunately, from the perspective of your child's health, British culture expects a hot meal to be followed by a pudding, so many schools will offer this, but there should also be a selection of fresh fruit available. Work through the menu with your child to help them make the best choices. If their choices are guided by someone at the nursery or school, then speak to that person, too. Overall, unless your child has specific dietary needs, a cooked meal at lunchtime is likely to be the best option and in some cases taking in a packed lunch is not permitted or will make your child feel 'different'. If the menu doesn't impress, get involved (see chapter 23 for more on this).

## Packed lunch

The three main types of packed lunch are sandwiches, salad box or, for older children, a flask of something hot, all accompanied by a piece of fresh fruit.

## Sandwiches

Sandwiches are the most straightforward to prepare and for your child to eat. Heavy, grainy bread with a protein and vegetable filling is ideal. For example, chicken, lettuce and tomato; hummus, red pepper and leaves; egg and cress. Even a peanut butter sandwich works if it's supplemented with some carrot or celery sticks. Raw veg alongside any sandwich makes a particularly good packed lunch and, as well as carrot and celery, you can include cherry tomatoes, baby corn, sugar snaps, strips of red, yellow or orange pepper, purple sprouting broccoli, and cauliflower or broccoli florets. They all work very well with a hummus dip, too.

If your child is avoiding gluten, then sandwiches will be off the menu, because good gluten-free bread needs toasting, but wraps made from 100 per cent corn tortillas, filled with sandwich fillings as above, work well.

## The salad box

A salad box will need protein, carbs and some veg in the ideal ratio of 1:1:2. Most parents find that the easiest way to prepare this type of packed lunch is to base it on the previous evening's meal. The main advantage of this is that it saves having to spend a lot of time putting the lunch box together in the morning, so, for example, if you're making pasta in the evening, cook a little extra and it becomes the base for a pasta salad lunch the next day. A dinner of salmon, brown rice, green beans and broccoli means it's cold salmon, rice salad (just add olive oil and lemon juice or balsamic vinegar) and some raw or lightly steamed green beans and broccoli in the lunch box the next day. Cold starchy vegetables such as potatoes and sweet potatoes can also be eaten as a potato salad – just add a mayonnaise or vinaigrette dressing. If your child is really not keen on using a fork at lunchtime, then try to make as much of the lunch out of finger food as possible. Sausage, meatballs, falafels, smoked mackerel, roast potatoes or parsnips and raw veg are all good examples.

## *The flask*

A flask of hot soup or stew can be a nutritious, warming lunch, which is particularly welcome in winter. As ever, you're aiming for the usual 1:1:2 proportions of protein, carbs and veg. This could be a spiced lentil, vegetable and rice soup, a traditional beef and veg stew complete with potato, parsnip and swede, or minestrone with plenty of kidney or aduki beans for protein. A chunk of wholemeal bread can accompany a soup that is light on the carbs.

# The evening meal

At the risk of repeating ourselves, again, you're aiming for the usual protein, carbs and veg proportions of 1:1:2.

The protein might be fish (especially an oily fish such as salmon, mackerel, trout or sardines), organic or free-range meat or eggs, or pulses. Lentils and beans may not be a food you grew up with, but they certainly deserve a prominent place in your family's diet. A great source of protein, they also add fibre and important nutrients, help hormonal balance and are economical to boot – helping offset some of the costs you may incur through buying organic, for instance. As cultures from India to Mexico know, they're also delicious and wonderfully versatile to cook with. You can use them to enliven a massive range of soups, stew, salads, veggieburgers, veggie dips and sandwich fillings – the list is endless.

Lentils are cooked from dry in a mere 15 to 30 minutes, depending on the variety. Beans and chickpeas can be bought in tins from any supermarket (look for those packed in water, without sugar or salt) and just need rinsing before use. Or if you're really keen you can buy them dried, soak overnight and boil for the time indicated on the packet. Note that pulses need to be chewed thoroughly, though, as otherwise they can cause gas.

All pulses apart from the 'split' kind can also be sprouted, making a tasty and amazingly nutritious addition to salads and sandwiches. As the sprouting process only takes three or four days, your child might enjoy growing their own food and experiencing the excitement of watching its progress, day by day.

Alongside the protein and unrefined carbs, such as brown rice, wholegrain pasta, potatoes or other starchy veg, the vegetable section should then include non-starchy vegetables, such as courgettes, broccoli, carrots, peppers, peas, tomatoes, onions and so on. These proportions persist whether the food is mixed together into one complete meal, such as a bean and vegetable stew, or whether the food sits separately on the plate, as in the case of a roast chicken dinner.

If a favourite meal doesn't quite fit the bill, then try adapting it so that it does. For example, pasta with a tomato-based sauce is a favourite for many children. On its own it lacks the protein and the vegetables to make it a complete meal. For the protein, add a tin of beans, some boiled lentils or make it a Bolognese by adding mince. The vegetables can be added in a number of ways. If your children won't eat obvious vegetables, blend them up and hide them in the sauce. Otherwise, you can add the chopped vegetables to the sauce. Another option is to provide the raw vegetables or a salad as a first course for your child to eat while you're preparing the meal.

Adapting their favourites applies whether it's a shepherd's pie or a roast dinner. For instance, it's rare to find real gravy served with a roast dinner these days, but this is a real shame, as gravy made the old-fashioned way, from thickened meat juice, has a wonderful natural flavour compared to the chemically enhanced flavour of instant gravy and it really is quick to make – use cornflour as the thickener and it's gluten-free! For the vegetarians, our favourite is red onion gravy. Make it by gently sautéing diced red onions and thickening with vegetable bouillon powder. Marigold's vegetable bouillon comes in several varieties, is gluten-free, contains no chemical additives and is widely available in supermarkets.

Finally, if you want to give soups, stews and curries a rich, creamy touch, you don't have to go for cream, as creamed coconut, coconut milk or a dab of hummus or tahini are healthy, dairy-free options.

## Choosing fats and oils for cooking

If you must fry, far and away the best cooking oil is coconut. Despite its lardy appearance at fridge or room temperature, coconut oil is a very healthy choice, because it cannot be harmed by heating. The medium-chain triglycerides or MCTs it contains are also much easier for the body to burn for energy, so it's less likely to be stored as fat. And don't worry – it has virtually no flavour of its own. The next best option is butter, unless you're dairy-free, followed by olive oil (a monounsaturated fat), which is slightly damaged by frying.

Whichever you use, never fry on a high heat. Instead, steam-fry, as the temperature and nutrient loss are much lower with this method. With onions and garlic, for instance, sauté them in your chosen oil so that you generate some heat and soften them slightly; then add the other ingredients and a dash of water, stock or soy sauce. Clamp the lid on and steam gently for a few minutes until they're cooked through.

# Snacks

Children need snacks to keep their blood sugar levels even and their energy levels up. Ideally, they'll snack mid-morning and mid-afternoon. The best and easiest snacks are fresh fruit with some fresh seeds and nuts. The fruit provides the carbohydrates and antioxidant vitamins, while the seeds and nuts provide protein, essential fats and minerals. Toasted seeds are almost as healthy as fresh. You can make delicious home-made toasted pumpkin seeds with a dash of tamari or there are a number of toasted varieties available from health food shops and some supermarkets.

Raw vegetables are a super-nutritious snack, and are especially nice with hummus or other bean dips. Vegetables such as sugar snaps and cherry tomatoes are great for kids, because they can

help themselves directly from the fridge and there's no preparation required, plus you don't need to be concerned about them
ruining their appetite for tea if they're eating raw vegetables or
fruit!

Many children are very hungry at the end of the school day. It's
understandable – their brains have been working hard all day. If
you find that these healthy snacks don't sustain them until the
evening meal and they're getting through half a loaf of bread without pausing for breath, consider bringing the meal forward, if
that's possible, or providing some more sustaining healthy snacks,
such as a bowl of chunky soup.

Some other snacks, which might be seen as reasonably healthy,
are plain popcorn and rice cakes, although these have a rather high
GL and so should be accompanied by some protein. Cereals bars
and flapjacks also tend to have a high GL, and, although they do
make a convenient snack, they shouldn't be eaten too often.

## Drinks

Without a doubt, water is the best staple drink for children. It's a
sign of the times that many children will not even consider water
as an option for a drink unless there's absolutely nothing else and
they're desperately thirsty! In these days of the childhood obesity
epidemic and rising levels of diabetes in children, our advice is to
steer clear of the empty calories and concentrated sugar found in
most drinks, particularly those aimed at children. As with adults,
children will be happy with water if that's what they're used to,
leaving room for an occasional juice or even a fizzy drink as a
treat.

There's an old adage in nutrition – good food goes off. The best
juices are those that have a very short shelf-life, because those
juices won't have been treated to keep them 'fresh'. Diluting them
with water is advisable and, if your child is used to drinking water,
they'll find them too sweet if they drink them neat anyway. Don't

be tempted by the declarations of 'sugar-free' or 'diet' on the labels. What this means is that the drink contains a synthetic sugar substitute, most likely aspartame, which may be associated with worrying side-effects and certainly doesn't improve the nutritional value of the product.

## Two-day menu

**Breakfast**
Porridge with chopped plums and seeds

**Snack**
An apple and a handful of raw cashews

**Lunch**
Spaghetti Bolognese with pureed vegetables hidden in the sauce

**Snack**
Sugar snap peas and cherry tomatoes

**Dinner**
Fish, mashed potatoes, broccoli and French beans

**Drinks throughout the day**
Diluted fresh fruit juice or water

**Breakfast**
Wholegrain toast with almond butter

**Snack**
A pear and some pumpkin seeds

**Lunch**
Pasta shapes with a chicken and tomato sauce
Carrot and celery sticks

**Snack**
Oat biscuits and a plum

**Dinner**
Stew with chickpeas and a variety of vegetables

**Drinks throughout the day**
Diluted fresh fruit juice or water

# The 80:20 rule

For most children, the 80:20 rule applies. This means that provided they eat healthily for 80 per cent of the time, you can relax for the other 20 per cent. While you can provide your child with healthy food at home, keeping this up can be difficult when they visit friends or go to parties, or when your family eats out or goes on holiday, but as long as their basic diet is the best it can be, the occasional packet of crisps or bowl of chocolate ice cream is fine. What's more, if you explain that there's one way of eating at home and another way of eating elsewhere, you can help your child associate these 'treats' with special occasions and not pester you for them all the time. However, it's wise not to make this a big issue or your child will begin to see certain foods as 'forbidden' and this will just enhance their appeal, especially if they can see that you view these foods as 'forbidden naughty treats' for yourself as well. Be blasé when you're eating that bowl of ice cream!

The exceptions to the 80:20 rule are children who have more complex or severe health problems, such as autism or life-threatening food allergies. For these children a stricter approach may be necessary for a period of at least a year or two, or in some cases for life.

## Summary

To provide an ideal diet for your child:

- Make every meal and snack count towards nourishing your child. Choose fresh, whole foods every time.

- Always combine protein with carbohydrate for good blood sugar balance. Meals should be 25 per cent protein-rich foods, 25 per cent carbohydrate-rich foods and 50 per cent non-starchy vegetables. That's a ratio of 1:1:2.

- Regular, healthy snacks are important for children.

# Chapter 23

# Finding the end of the rainbow

Now you know what the pot of gold looks like, let's set off to find it! If your child has developed a taste for less-than-healthy foods, you'll need to change their diet. Does the mere idea fill you with foreboding? Don't worry. Although it can be tough weaning them off double-cheese pizzas and chips with everything, this chapter shows it can be done gradually and relatively painlessly.

No matter where your child's diet is at or what their age, what you need to know is that now is the time to start the journey towards optimum nutrition for your child. Whatever age your child is now, improving their diet will only be more difficult the older they get as they become more set in their ways and independent. It will almost certainly be challenging, but we have lots of tricks up our sleeves to help you move your child along.

Before you begin, let's talk about the project. In the same way as building an extension to your house is a project, improving your child's diet is a project, too. First, you need to know what your aims are, and we outlined those in the previous chapter. Next, you need to make a plan. If you're getting the builders in, there are certain things you have to do before they arrive. For example, you need to plan the sequence of events, so that when the plumber turns up to install the kitchen, the kitchen units are already on site and so on. During the project there may be times when you can't see the wood for the trees, but in the end, when you've achieved your goal, you'll barely remember the disruption as you stand back and appreciate the results of your efforts.

In the same way, you need to plan the project of improving your child's diet. Your child's diet may need a few minor tweaks or you might be looking at a major overhaul, but either way, you'll need to identify what changes need to be made, what the priorities are and what you're going to tackle first.

## CASE HISTORY *Jerome, age 4*

Jerome was brought to see us at the Brain Bio Centre with language delay and other difficulties such as nervousness, hypersensitivity to noise, lack of interaction with others and mild constipation. His mother was aware that children do better on a healthy diet, but despite her best efforts, Jerome ate almost nothing other than crackers, pancakes, cheese, ice cream and baked beans. He had a real aversion to new foods.

Our initial aim was to broaden the range of foods that Jerome would eat. We started by recommending that his mum make up an ice cube tray of pureed red pepper and carrot, and added half a teaspoon of this mixture to his baked beans, gradually increasing the amount over time. We also suggested adding some pureed fruit to his ice cream and, as Jerome would only eat vanilla flavour ice cream, we suggested fresh pear and melon because we were looking for a colour match.

When new foods were put on Jerome's plate, we also asked his mother to keep a list of the ones that Jerome would either touch, lick, nibble or eat. Initially, just touching a new food was a real achievement. Over time with patient encouragement, he would pick up a new food, lick it and put it back down. Gradually, over a period of months, foods slowly moved from 'will lick' to 'will nibble' column and then over to the 'will eat' column on the list.

Meanwhile, the baked beans had evolved into a mixed bean and vegetable stew and the ice cream had developed into a pureed fruit and seed blend. It took many months and a huge effort by Jerome's family, but now he eats quite a variety of foods. He also has a much greater vocabulary, better concentration, more confidence, greater participation and regular bowel movements. His parents are really thrilled with the results and Jerome has even developed an interest in trying new foods!

Jerome's case is extreme, but it demonstrates that even children who are on severely self-restricted diets can learn to develop a taste for a wide range of foods. Making the changes can take a lot of time and patience, and if you're child is underweight, bordering on underweight, or their health is fragile, you'll need to ensure they at least maintain their weight throughout this process. Consequently, you may have to make the changes at an even slower pace.

## Make a plan

Start by getting a lever arch folder and labelling it with an inspiring title. This is now your project workbook. Then visit our website and have a look at the child's diet transformation pack at www.foodforthebrain.org/. In this pack, you'll find various items, including a diet diary sheet, and documents headed 'My aims for my child', 'My child's aims' and 'Areas to improve', as well as the template for a star chart. Print out those that are appropriate for your child and file them in your folder.

### My aims for my child

Make a detailed list of the reasons you want to improve your child's diet. For example, it might be to address particular health problems such as eczema or sleep problems, or to improve your child's health prospects, behaviour or school performance.

## My child's aims

Depending on the age of your child, you should also discuss with them some of their dreams and aspirations. Your child may want to do better in school, have more friends, be a faster runner or a better football player. Getting your child working with you, rather than against you, from the earliest possible age, is really helpful.

## Diet diary

Keep a food diary for your child. Ensure it includes samples of different days, such as nursery/school days, weekends and a regular day out with their grandparents. If they have a tendency towards being underweight, make a note of their weight so you can keep a check on it.

## Areas to improve

Compare your child's diet with what we've outlined in the previous chapter and identify the weaknesses in your child's diet. This might include such things as 'eats no fruit', 'only eats white bread', 'not enough protein with the evening meal' and so on. Write down as many as you can.

## Prioritise

Start by deciding which aspects of your child's diet you're going to tackle first. Depending on your child and your particular set of circumstances, you may decide to tackle a number of aims at once or target just one aspect of your child's diet, but be specific by setting objectives such as 'eat wholegrain bread at home and at school', 'eat two vegetables every day' or 'eat breakfast every day'.

## Map out the steps

For your chosen priorities, map out the steps that you and your child are going to take to achieve your objectives. This might be 'switch to a mixed white/brown loaf for one month, then switch to brown for one month, then switch to wholegrain'. On vegetables, it might be 'begin with blended vegetables in pasta sauce, gradually making them chunkier over time'. Or you could opt for 'eat a carrot stick, cherry tomato, or sugar snap every day before tea, increasing to two'.

## Do the groundwork

Get the whole family on board if you can. This means older siblings, grandparents, and so on. If they can't be convinced to be helpful, then at least get their agreement not to sabotage your efforts. Talk to everyone who is involved with food, education and your child. Find out what happens at nursery. If all the children get a beaker of 'juice', can yours have a beaker of diluted juice or water? Nobody wants their child to feel different, but most beakers are opaque, so your child's peers won't notice. What do they feed the children? Do the children get to make any choices? If you're not happy with what's on offer at nursery or school, do something about it (see chapter 24 for more on this).

## Clear the cupboards

Clear the cupboards and get rid of as much of the rubbish as possible. If might be fun to conduct a 'cleansing ceremony' as you dispatch the junk to its rightful place in the bin or perhaps you could have a 'final feast of filth' where everyone fills up on the junk to the point of nausea. Relocate those decadent dessert recipes books to the top shelf and invest in some healthier recipe books (see Recommended reading). Then go shopping and stock up on some healthy staples (see Shopping list).

# Strategies to employ

Now you're ready to start. You may well have to use all your wit and guile to change your child's eating habits, but it will be worth it. Use your project workbook to keep track of your progress and look back at it from time to time, to remind yourself how far you've actually come.

## Lead by example

This is probably the most important strategy to adopt. It may seem obvious, but we've worked with many families where the parents are struggling to get their children to eat vegetables and yet one or other of the parent eats none.

## Manage choices

By clearing the cupboards you are already managing your child's choices. The simple answer to 'why can't I have sugar puffs for breakfast?' is a clear and concise 'because we don't have any'. When offering a meal or snack, don't ask an open question, such as 'what would you like to eat?' Instead, ask a conveniently closed question, such as 'would you like an apple or an orange?' or 'do you want pasta or fish for tea?'

## Encouragement and enthusiasm

It's vitally important that mealtimes don't become running battles or times of stress. To keep them relatively peaceful you'll probably have to adapt your strategies as you go along, but that's part of the process. If one strategy isn't working, try something else.

## Consider the family dynamics

Is Johnny a real daddy's boy or will Jill do anything for grandma? If this is the case, make the most it. Johnny's father can show his son how to eat vegetables to make him big and strong, while an extra visit to grandma might be all that Jill needs to persuade her to eat her greens.

## Are there emotional issues?

Sometimes an educational or child psychologist can provide expert advice tailored to your child's personality and this can be invaluable in getting over that first hump. Perhaps your child already has a learning support assistant or is following a specific educational programme? If so, make the most of that and ensure that any extra help your child receives is reinforcing the message on good food. For example, non-verbal autistic children are often taught to use picture card systems to make requests for food, so ensure that the food cards are consistent with your aims.

## Charts and stars

Star charts and stickers work brilliantly for many young children. Develop the chart and the rules together with your child, so that they 'buy into' the system. Our child's diet transformation pack includes a template which you can enlarge and laminate or you could make your own. Here's an example:

| Food | Sun | Mon | Tues | Wed | Thurs | Fri | Sat | **TOTAL** |
|---|---|---|---|---|---|---|---|---|
| 1 green vegetable | ✓ | ✓ | ✓ | ✓ | ✓ | ✓ | ✓ | |
| 1 fruit | ✓ | ✓ | ✗ | ✓ | ✓ | ✓ | ✓ | |
| 5 pumpkin seeds | ✓ | ✓ | ✓ | ✓ | ✓ | ✓ | ✓ | |
| **TOTAL** | ✓ | ✓ | ✗ | ✓ | ✓ | ✓ | ✓ | ✗ |

7 ticks = football with dad on Sunday

You can make the chart colourful and fun by drawing pictures of particular foods, cutting photos out of magazines and, in some cases, actually gluing the food to the chart! A young daughter might respond best to a fairy that moves up a rainbow with a prize for reaching the top. The prize might be a new arts and crafts set that you can use together to make a new chart. The next time it could be a flower with petals added for trying a new food, with a prize awarded when the flower is complete. Your young son might like a train that moves along a track, with prizes being given out each time the train reaches a station. Try to tap in to what will work best for your child, and above all make sure that a small failure doesn't make it impossible to win the reward. For some children, just putting one mouthful of a new food into their mouth is a big step. Even if they decide they don't like it, don't give up on it. Just serve it up again another time – eventually, with a few possible exceptions, they will be happy to eat it.

Another way of incentivising good eating behaviour is by handing out coloured poker chips during meals. At the end of the week, the child can cash them in with you, either for money or for something else. Alternatively, they could keep them until they've filled up a jar, which has a picture on it of the prize they'll get when the jar is full, such as a new toy or a trip to London.

Always remember that you're on your child's side. Your child can see on the chart that they only have to put one forkful of peas in their mouth to get today's sticker, so be disappointed for them if they can't manage it and excited for them if they do. You want them to have the sticker, but the rules are the rules.

## Play hide and seek

If your child refuses to eat vegetables, but will eat tomato sauce, begin by adding small amounts of pureed vegetables to the sauce and increase the amount, teaspoon by teaspoon, over the days and weeks. This way, they simply won't notice the changing taste and appearance, but within three months their tastebuds will have become used to the vegetables and they'll actually be eating a highly nutritious, vitamin-rich sauce with their pasta. After this, it's simply a case of blending the vegetables less and less thoroughly, so they get chunkier over time. When you finally present a plate of vegetables to your child, their tastebuds will register them as a familiar food and they are more likely to actually enjoy eating them.

## Make your own healthier versions

For children who will only eat fish fingers and chicken nuggets, begin by making your own, but try to make them look similar to the commercial varieties. You can begin to add pureed steamed vegetables, pureed boiled lentils or pureed beans to these fish or chicken mixtures, too. Add tiny amounts at the start, then increase gradually. Eventually, your child will be eating lentil and vegetable fingers and burgers that are rich in nutrients and fibre, instead of packaged food that may be of dubious quality and devoid of nutrients.

## Treat the tastebuds

One of the biggest problems with getting children who eat a lot of junk food to switch to healthy wholefoods is the powerful artificial flavours and additives lurking in so many highly processed products. At the start, wholefoods can seem bland by comparison, but perseverance, the gradual introduction of healthy ingredients as outlined above, and a clever use of herbs, spices, nutritious oils, lemon juice and the like can work wonders. For example, steamed vegetables can be served with a squeeze of lemon juice, a dollop of hummus, a knob of butter, a vinaigrette dressing, fresh salsa and so on.

## Special cups and plates

Research shows that how food is presented to children has a considerable influence over whether they will like it. Consider this study of 46 children aged from three to six. They each tasted ten flavours, half of which were presented in a positive way, while the other half were not. Then the children were given the flavours a second time without differences in presentation and randomly interspersed with ten more flavours. The children aged four and a half and older were better able to identify, and liked the taste more, of the five flavours that had originally had the positive presentation.[1]

This means that if you want your child to eat a boiled egg for breakfast, take them to a crockery painting shop and have them paint their own egg cup. You can make or paint all sorts of other crockery, too – perhaps a special dinner plate that is divided into sections for the proteins, carbs and veg?

## Get the children involved

Research by the British Food Council shows that children are more willing to eat the food they themselves have chosen. So while you need to keep this simple to avoid overwhelming your child or even encouraging fussiness, you can involve them more as they grow. For example, ask them to pick out some fruit and vegetables in the supermarket, or get them involved in preparing meals. They can begin by sprinkling sunflower seeds on a salad and work their way up to helping prepare complete meals. Many kids like baking cakes with mum at the weekend. Make sure you choose healthier recipes. And there's no reason why you can't make healthy meals rather than baking sweet treats.

## Growing food

Research shows that children eat more vegetables if they're home-grown, especially if they're also involved in cultivating those vegetables. It can be thrilling for children to observe the daily growth of plants and fun for them to harvest food from the garden. You might not have the space for a veggie patch, but a window box will suffice. Sprouting is another fun way to get your children interested in eating all sorts of sprouts. Most seeds and pulses take only a few days until they're ready to eat (see Recommended reading and Products and supplements directory for more on this).

## Everyone has their price

Money talks and if nothing else will convince your child to ditch the junk, you might have to resort to paying them, although you'll need to work out a system, with firm rules as to exactly how much they get and for what. Again, keep things visible and fun, though. Make up a thermometer-style chart on the wall, like the ones used by schools and other fund-raisers, or get a tall basket that can be filled with plastic balls, with different prizes that can be won at different heights, as children need short-term and long-term goals. Younger children will also need daily goals that add up to weekly targets, whereas older children will do better with weekly and monthly targets.

## Good old-fashioned discipline

Your grandparents and possibly even your own parents would not have stood for their children refusing to eat and they wouldn't have hesitated to send an errant child to bed without supper. If you make the threat, be prepared to carry it out. If your child chooses not to eat their dinner at all, cover the plate and put it to one side. Later, if your child complains of hunger, offer to reheat it for them. If you allow them to fill up on toast, because you can't bear the idea of them being hungry, they will have won. However, clearly you need to use your discretion, as this method is not suitable for children who are underweight or have serious issues with food.

# Eating outside the home

Once your child starts attending nursery or school, or spends time in other types of childcare, your control over their diet begins to slip away, but you still need to take a strong interest in what your child is eating when you're not around.

## At nursery or school

It's particularly important to check out nurseries, because young children aren't really able to make choices about food themselves. Before you commit to one, find out what they will feed your child. If it doesn't impress, look elsewhere. If parents demand better food for their children, nurseries will provide it.

At school, however, what a child eats is likely to be completely up to them. If your child already has an appetite for healthy food, then they are more likely to make healthy choices. If not, then it is doubly important that the choices on offer are good.

When working with children who choose their own lunch at school, we find that it's important for them to have a good incentive to eat healthily. A lower risk of heart disease in later life is unlikely to impress a ten-year-old, but if you tell them it will help them be a better football player, do better in class, stop getting into trouble and have clear skin, that's much more motivating. Optimum nutrition improves health and well-being on a myriad of levels, but you need to focus on what's important to your child. After all, being better at maths is not much of an incentive to an artistic child who has no interest in maths.

## Breakfast clubs

These clubs are theoretically a great idea, but if you need to use this service, you'll have to take a hard look at what's on the menu first. If 'breakfast' is sugary cereal, white toast, jam and juice drinks, you're effectively putting your child on a blood sugar rollercoaster, so you have two options: exert your influence as a concerned parent to ensure that better breakfasts are available or give your child breakfast at home.

## On the way to and from school

Once your child has their own money, and is walking to and from school on their own, you can't stop them from buying sweets at the shop on the way. However, if their schoolbag is full of healthy snacks and their pockets are not weighted down with cash, you will have less to worry about. Also, if they've had a good breakfast at home, they'll be less inclined to buy food on the journey to school, and if they're used to nutritious, wholesome food and have balanced blood sugar, they will be less inclined to gorge on the really unhealthy stuff. Try not to make too big a deal about this, though, as on the whole the food your child eats will be what you provide for them at home and that is what's most important.

## Carers and relatives

In an ideal world, anyone who spends any time with your child will embrace optimum nutrition as you do, but if yours is not an ideal world you may need to give them some guidance. If you're paying a carer to look after your child, you simply need to give them clear instructions and an explanation, so they understand why you want them to feed your child some foods and not others.

If your child spends time with grandparents or other relatives, a lot more diplomacy is needed. Older people are more often set in their ways and many will like to treat their grandchildren when they see them. If visits are rare, then this isn't a problem, but if they're frequent you may need to tactfully talk through with them the reasons behind your food choices for your child and ask for their cooperation. In all cases, you might need to consider providing some food.

## The dreaded children's menu

In many restaurants, the children's menu features the most unhealthy food on the entire menu – typically a burger, fries, ice cream and a fizzy drink. The restaurant industry insists that they are simply offering customers choice, so it's up to customers to vote with their feet. You don't have to order food from the children's menu at all. Order an adult starter, share a main dish with your child, ask for a steamed vegetable or salad to be substituted for the chips and opt for diluted juices instead of fizzy drinks. However, remember the 80:20 rule. As long as your child eats healthily 80 per cent of the time, you don't have to worry unduly for the other 20 per cent, so the occasional unhealthy meal won't hurt.

## Summary

To help your child change their diet:

- Identify what you want to achieve and why, and make a plan.

- Use a range of strategies to persuade your child to eat more healthily. Older children do best if they have a clear understanding of how they benefit.

- Take as much control of your child's diet outside the home as you can, but remember the 80:20 rule and don't be too rigid all the time.

# Chapter 24

•

# Guerrilla tactics in the supermarket

You'll have to face it sooner or later – what you want for your child, and what the food manufacturers and marketeers want, are two different things. This means you need to develop guerrilla tactics in the supermarket, reading the labels carefully – and reading between the lines. The hopeful news is that, these days, there really is plenty of choice, even in mainstream supermarkets. Add in what health food stores have to offer and it just isn't that difficult to fill cupboard and fridge with wonderfully nutritious and delicious foods.

Here are the 12 golden rules for shopping:

## Avoid foods that contain hydrogenated fats

Check the label for the words 'hydrogenated' and 'vegetable oil'. If it contains vegetable oil and has a long shelf-life, the oil in the product has been hydrogenated – that is, processed so that it hardens. As we discussed in chapter 3, hydrogenated fats interfere with the brain's use of essential fats and, ultimately, with the smooth working of the brain.

## Avoid foods that contain sugar

Check the label for sugar. This includes honey, syrup, sucrose, glucose, dextrose, maltose and any other '-ose'. Sugars that won't play havoc with your child's blood glucose include xylitol, fructose and blue agave syrup, which is used in drinks, but only go for products where even these sugars are a long way down the ingredient list.

## Avoid processed juice and fruit juice drinks

As discussed in chapter 1, processed fruit juices and fruit juice drinks are no better than sugary water. With these products, don't be fooled by the manufacturer's assertion that the drink has been fortified with vitamins and minerals. All this means is that the original and natural nutrients have been destroyed through processing. The only acceptable juices are freshly made ones or the kind that's kept in the chill cabinet and has a very short shelf-life – just a few days, maximum. Apple juice is the best choice, since apples contain mainly fructose.

## Buy small blocks of cheese and small cartons of milk

Consuming a lot of dairy products can potentially trigger a sensitivity to these foods – after all, milk is one of the top allergens. Most cheese also has a lot of saturated fat. If you and your children are eating dairy products, don't buy family-sized blocks of cheese and 5 litre containers of milk – unless you are a family of 20! Buying smaller packages will keep your consumption down to a moderate level. Buy stronger-flavoured cheese, such as Parmesan or mature Cheddar, so that it can be used as a garnish rather than be eaten by the slab.

## Choose free-range, organic and omega-3 rich eggs

Eggs are a superb food, but they're only as healthy as the chicken who laid them. If you can, buy omega-3 enriched eggs, preferably organic or at least free-range.

## Avoid foods that contain additives, preservatives and other chemicals

Check the list of unacceptable additives and avoid these rigorously (see chapter 6), but familiarise yourself with the much shorter list of healthy E numbers, which are actually vitamins, too (see chapter 6 again). As a good rule of thumb, a shorter ingredient list is likely to indicate a healthier food. For example, bread may have as few as three ingredients or as many as 30. Most importantly, if you read a long ingredient list and don't recognise many of these substances as 'food' – that is, something that grew on a tree or in the ground, for example – or you feel you could better recognise and pronounce them if you had a chemistry degree, this should sound the alarm bells that this product is not a good thing to give your child.

## Make a list and stick to it

This is especially important if your child is going to the supermarket with you. You could write the list together. Use generic terms such as 'fruit and veg' so you're not limiting yourself and can pick what looks good. Don't put anything in the trolley that's not on the list, unless of course it's something you genuinely forgot you needed (and that clearly doesn't include chocolate biscuits!). If you're strict about this your child will accept it. Never cave in to your child's demands and don't be frightened of a tantrum. Caving in teaches them that a tantrum gets them exactly what they want. Avoid the biscuits and sweets aisle altogether. Remember, if they watch children's TV, every ad break is showcasing some refined, sugar-laden food that comes with a small plastic gift. Stay away from them!

## Eat before you go shopping

If your child is coming with you, give them a snack, too. An apple and a few Brazil nuts in the car on the way to the supermarket will keep their blood sugar levels even. This deflects their cravings for sugary foods and also prevents the irritability that goes along with it. Take a drink of water into the supermarket, too.

## Buy organic when you can

Sometimes there is very little price difference between organic and non-organic foods, which is a boon, but be careful about organic processed foods. The ingredients are probably better quality, and it's likely to be E number-free, but organic pizza and chips are still pizza and chips, and organic cake can still be laden with sugar. And as we've seen, refined carbohydrates add nothing to a healthy diet.

## Choose whole foods over refined and processed

This means brown rice, wholemeal pasta, and wholegrain bread instead of white. Choose whole vegetables, not ready-prepared vegetables – these will have been haemorrhaging nutrients since they were sliced. It's better, and much cheaper, to buy a whole lettuce or cabbage than to buy prepared salads or salad greens that go off within minutes of opening the bag.

## Variety is the spice of life

Be adventurous and try new things, especially fresh produce and pulses. Have you ever eaten quinoa or pearl barley, or had grated beetroot raw in a salad? Variety is key to good nutrition and makes mealtimes a lot more pleasurable, too.

## Watch out for '95% fat free'

As we discussed in chapter 3, fat phobia is misguided. It's the *type* of fat that counts. Most products that claim to be low fat have had sugar added to make them palatable, so they're not any better than the original. In fact, they're probably worse. Watch out for reduced-fat items, where the original item is actually a naturally high-fat food. An example is low-fat butter. The point about butter is that it's supposed to be virtually 100 per cent fat, so check the ingredient list to see what's been added instead.

# Chapter 25

·

# Supplements for superkids

We've demonstrated throughout this book that a varied and nutritious diet is the keystone of good health – physical, mental and emotional – for your child. However, sometimes even the best diets fail to provide appropriate levels of all the nutrients we need – food often travels from afar and may have been stored for months, children can be very picky eaters, and so on. Due to their biological uniqueness, some children may also have a greater need for certain nutrients. Add to all this the logistical challenge of providing a day's meals perfectly balanced in every nutrient and what you're looking at is supplements.

Supplementation is the most reliable way to ensure your child gets appropriate levels of all the vitamins and minerals they need to be optimally nourished. This is even more important if your child has health challenges, whether that be from frequent infections, or behavioural or sleep problems. Remember that there's a range of vitamins and minerals essential for good health, and a small deficiency in any one nutrient could have an impact on your growing child.

# When to start supplementing

As soon as you start weaning your child, it's worth supplementing. As long as you're breast-feeding, it's you that needs to take the supplemental nutrients, which then get passed on to them naturally.

The chart below shows the ideal daily amounts of vitamins, minerals and essential fats to supplement from weaning to age 13, assuming you're also feeding them a reasonably healthy diet. Once a child is 14, adult levels of nutrients apply, which you can find in *The Optimum Nutrition Bible* by Patrick Holford or the optimum daily allowances tables at www.patrickholford.com.

## THE IDEAL DAILY SUPPLEMENT PROGRAMME

| Age | Less than 1 | 1–2 | 3–4 | 5–6 | 7–8 | 9–11 | 12–13 |
|---|---|---|---|---|---|---|---|
| **Nutrient** | | | | | | | |
| *Vitamins* | | | | | | | |
| A (retinol) (mcg) | 500 | 650 | 800 | 1000 | 1500 | 2000 | 2500 |
| D (mcg) | 3 | 4 | 5 | 7 | 9 | 11 | 12 |
| E (mg) | 13 | 16 | 20 | 23 | 30 | 40 | 50 |
| C (mg) | 100 | 150 | 300 | 400 | 500 | 600 | 700 |
| B1 (thiamine) (mg) | 5 | 6 | 8 | 12 | 16 | 20 | 24 |
| B2 (riboflavin) (mg) | 5 | 6 | 8 | 12 | 16 | 20 | 24 |
| B3 (niacin) (mg) | 7 | 12 | 16 | 18 | 20 | 22 | 24 |
| B5 (pantothenic acid) (mg) | 10 | 15 | 20 | 25 | 30 | 35 | 40 |
| B6 (pyridoxine) (mg) | 5 | 7 | 10 | 12 | 16 | 20 | 25 |
| B12 (mcg) | 5 | 6.5 | 8 | 9 | 10 | 10 | 10 |
| Folic acid (mcg) | 100 | 120 | 140 | 160 | 180 | 200 | 220 |
| Biotin (mcg) | 30 | 45 | 60 | 70 | 80 | 90 | 100 |
| *Minerals* | | | | | | | |
| Calcium (mg) | 150 | 165 | 180 | 190 | 200 | 210 | 220 |
| Magnesium (mg) | 50 | 65 | 80 | 90 | 100 | 110 | 120 |
| Iron (mg) | 4 | 5.5 | 7 | 8 | 9 | 10 | 10 |
| Zinc (mg) | 4 | 5.5 | 7 | 8 | 9 | 10 | 10 |

continues →

| Age | Less than 1 | 1–2 | 3–4 | 5–6 | 7–8 | 9–11 | 12–13 |
|---|---|---|---|---|---|---|---|
| Manganese (mcg) | 300 | 350 | 400 | 500 | 700 | 1000 | 1000 |
| Iodine (mcg) | 40 | 50 | 60 | 70 | 80 | 90 | 100 |
| Chromium (mcg) | 15 | 19 | 23 | 25 | 27 | 30 | 30 |
| Selenium (mcg) | 10 | 18 | 20 | 24 | 26 | 28 | 30 |
| Copper (mcg) | 400 | 550 | 700 | 800 | 900 | 1000 | 1000 |
| *Essential fats* | | | | | | | |
| GLA (mg) | 50 | 75 | 95 | 110 | 135 | 135 | 135 |
| EPA (mg) | 100 | 175 | 250 | 300 | 350 | 350 | 350 |
| DHA (mg) | 100 | 140 | 175 | 200 | 225 | 225 | 225 |

**Extra brain nutrients (optional – see part 2 for more on this)**

| | |
|---|---|
| Phosphatidyl choline (PC) (mg) | 250 to 400mg |
| Phosphatidyl serine (PS) (mg) | 20 to 45mg |
| DMAE (mg) | 200 to 300mg |
| Glutamine (mg) | 250 to 1000mg |
| (Arginine) pyroglutamate (mg) | 300 to 450mg |
| Trimethyl glycine (TMG) (mg) | 250mg–1000mg |

# Choosing the right supplements

With supplements for your child, you're looking at a multivitamin and mineral formula, plus essential fats. Children with specific emotional, learning or behavioural problems may benefit from extra brain nutrients as well.

## Finding a good multi

Many companies formulate single multivitamin and mineral supplements that incorporate all the necessary nutrients especially for children (see page 295). The chart above gives you guidelines on the levels of nutrients to look for. You can choose chewable (or crushable in the early stages), liquid or soluble formulas, depending on your child's preferences.

You should ideally give your child his or her supplement with breakfast, but certainly not last thing at night, as the B vitamins can have a mild stimulatory effect. (Glutamine can also be stimulating for some children, especially those on the autistic spectrum, for whom it may not be suitable.) Children also tend to be more susceptible to vitamin toxicity than adults and, while the doses listed are well within any potentially toxic limits for even the most sensitive child, don't be tempted to give much more than these recommended levels unless under the direction and supervision of a nutritional therapist.

You may notice that the levels of nutrients we recommend are considerably higher than the RDA. This is because the RDAs for most essential nutrients are defined as the amount required to prevent an overt deficiency disease. For example, the RDA for vitamin C is adequate to prevent scurvy, but there is plenty of evidence that the optimum intake to promote optimum health is several times higher than the RDA. Some essential nutrients, for example the essential fats, do not even have an RDA set for them.

Unless you're trying to correct a specific problem and giving glutamine powder or probiotics, in most cases you'll choose a chewable multivitamin and mineral, usually giving one for every two years of life. This means that by the time your child is eight they'll be taking four a day, although this does, of course, depend on the quantity of vitamins and minerals in the supplements, so check the levels against our guidelines. The supplements are best spread out, perhaps two with breakfast and two with lunch. If need be, you can always crush any supplement and add it to water or diluted fruit juice.

Few chewable multis contain enough vitamin C, zinc, calcium or magnesium, though. This is because vitamin C tastes tart, zinc tastes metallic, and calcium and magnesium make chewables crunchy – and less chewable! However, there are a number of ways round this problem. Assuming you are giving your child ground seeds every day, as we recommend, these will guarantee a reasonable amount of zinc, calcium and magnesium. You can get powdered calcium/magnesium to add to drinks, or a chewable vitamin C that uses calcium/magnesium ascorbate and zinc in drop form, also for adding to drinks, and this kills three birds with one stone. If your child doesn't sleep well, and a little extra magnesium would help, this is a good option. The best way to give your child a little extra vitamin C is to make sure they eat at least five servings of fruit and vegetables a day. The best foods for vitamin C are peppers, broccoli, berries and citrus fruit.

## Essential fats

As long as your child is eating oily fish three times a week and a daily portion of seeds, they should be getting a good background level of essential fats to help their brains develop, boost their IQ, support their immune system and keep their skin healthy. However, if they don't eat fish or don't have seeds every day, we recommend you supplement their diet with an essential fat formula. The chart gives you the rough quantities to aim for in a supplement, assuming they are receiving the same again from seeds and the occasional serving of oily fish, and look for one that contains both GLA (omega-6) and DHA and EPA, which are the most important omega-3 fats for development (see Products and supplements directory). The most important essential fat is omega-3 and there are many different forms of supplements on the market, ranging from gels to drinks to tiny capsules. You can always pierce a capsule and add it to juice or food.

## Extra brain nutrients

In addition to the essential vitamins, minerals and essential fats, we've also extolled the virtues of phospholipids (PC, PS and DMAE), as well as glutamine and its cousin pyroglutamate. These can be supplemented as well (see Products and supplements directory), but they usually come in tablets that may be hard for a younger child to swallow. For PC you can add some lecithin granules to cereal, generally giving a dessertspoon of regular lecithin or a teaspoonful of high-PC lecithin. Glutamine also comes in powder that easily dissolves in water or diluted juice.

## Summary

To ensure your child is getting enough nutrients:

- Give your child a good multivitamin and multimineral formula based on the nutrient levels given in this chapter.

- Give your child an omega-3 fish oil supplement with some omega-6 every day.

- If your child has emotional or behavioural challenges, look for a specific 'brain food' formula with the additional brain nutrients listed in this chapter and seek the advice of an experienced nutritional therapist.

# Shopping list

## Fruit and vegetables

**Fresh, low GL fruits** – apples, pears, plums, apricots, berries – preferably organic

**Frozen mixed berries** – berries have a very low GL and are full of bioflavonoids – frozen ones are a convenient way to include them in your child's diet all year round

**Fresh vegetables** – lettuce, rocket, watercress, spinach, cherry tomatoes, cucumber, spring onions, alfalfa sprouts, cress, courgettes, red onions, shallots, mushrooms, tenderstem, purple sprouting or normal broccoli, cabbage, aubergine, peppers and – preferably organic – ensure you choose plenty that can be eaten raw

**Baby new potatoes** – these have the lowest GL of all potatoes, as they are younger and smaller so have not developed such high sugar levels

**Sweet potatoes** – these are very rich in the antioxidant beta-carotene

**Fresh herbs** – basil, flat leaf parsley, coriander and chives

**Avocado** – a great low GL toast topping with a slice of tomato – or try adding olive oil, lemon juice, pepper and mashing with a fork – can include a clove of crushed garlic too if your child will eat it

**Lemons or limes** – ideal to squeeze on to fish to take the edge off the strong flavour

**Garlic**

**Fresh root ginger**

## Fresh products

**Organic milk** – or a dairy-free alternative such as soya, oat or quinoa milk – these all have a moderate GL, whereas rice and nut milks tend to have a high GL

**Live natural yoghurt** – or live sheep's or goat's yoghurt, which is more easily digested, or soya yoghurt, which is dairy-free

**Fresh or canned sardines, mackerel, pilchards and kippers (smoked herring)** – small oily fish like these accumulate less pollution and heavy metals than big carnivorous fish like tuna and swordfish, making them a safer source of omega-3 fish oils

## Store cupboard staples

**Organic and/or free-range eggs** – eggs from chickens fed on flaxseeds are a good source of omega-3 oils

**Dried or canned legumes and pulses** – lentils, chickpeas, borlotti, kidney, flageolet or mixed beans – choose ones canned in water or rinse thoroughly before use to remove as much salt from the canning liquid as possible

**Rye bread – pumpernickel-style or sourdough** – if your child is avoiding wheat check labels carefully as some brands add wheat

**Rough oat cakes** – rough ones have a nice coarse, chewy texture and a lower GL than finely milled varieties

**Wholemeal pasta** – choose a gluten-free variety such as brown rice or buckwheat pasta if necessary – buckwheat has a lower GL than rice or corn pasta

**Brown basmati rice** – has a nutty flavour, a chewy texture that's far more interesting than plain white rice and the lowest GL of all types of rice

**Soba noodles** – made from buckwheat, a gluten-free grain, these cook very quickly and can be used hot or cold in salads, steam fries or stir fries – look out for the 100 per cent buckwheat ones, as some brands also contain wheat

**Quinoa** – a delicious South American fruit, pronounced 'keen-wa', that looks and cooks like a grain (similar to rice) – contains all the essential amino acids, making it a perfect protein food that is also low in fat and rich in minerals – available in the speciality section of good supermarkets or from health food shops

**Whole organic oats** – available from good supermarkets and health food shops

**Whole barley and rye flakes** – can be used in place of oats, although they need slightly more cooking time – available from health food shops

**Cornflour** – for thickening sauces and puddings

**Coconut oil** – a very stable oil for cooking with – virtually flavourless and can be used for spreading, frying and baking – it's solid at room temperature and melts when heated to form an oil – will not raise cholesterol or produce harmful trans fats when cooked

**Extra virgin olive oil** – for salad dressings

**Sesame oil** – for Oriental dressings and dishes, and to enliven couscous, quinoa or rice salads

**Tamari** – wheat-free soy sauce – available from good supermarkets or health food shops – sprinkle on pumpkin seeds for home-toasting

**Canned chopped tomatoes** – cooked tomatoes contain more of the antioxidant lycopene than raw ones, making tomato products such as these useful and healthy

**Tomato purée**

**Sun-dried tomato paste**

**Jars of sauce** – good quality pasta and curry sauces are a great standby when you're short on time. Simply mix with lentils, beans or meat and some veg, and serve with wholegrain pasta or brown rice and you have a very quick, easy and healthy meal

**Olives** – avoid ones with colourings and additives – Greek Kalamata olives are wonderfully moist and full of flavour

**Pumpkin seed butter** – tastes very similar to peanut butter, but is richer in essential fats and zinc – a good alternative for most children with nut allergies – keep refrigerated after opening to protect the delicate omega-3 and 6 essential fats

**Crunchy peanut butter** – choose an unsweetened brand or another nut butter such as almond, hazelnut or cashew – the good ones list just two ingredients: the nut and salt

**Xylitol** – a naturally sweet, low-carb sugar alternative that doesn't disrupt blood sugar levels and has a third of the calories of sugar

**Unsalted, unroasted nuts and seeds** – for snacking and cooking

**Black peppercorns** – a light dusting on oily fish along with the lemon or lime juice helps to take the edge off the strong flavour

**Sea salt** – balanced in minerals and free from 'anti-caking agent'

**Vegetable bouillon powder** – a vegetarian, gluten-, yeast- and soya-free alternative to stock cubes – can be added to dishes at any stage of cooking as there's no need to dissolve it in water

**Dried herbs and spices** – look in health food shops for organic dried herbs and spices that have not been irradiated

# References

## Chapter 2: Not all carbohydrates are created equal

1   A. G. Schauss, 'Nutrition and behavior', *Journal of Applied Nutrition*, vol 35(1), pp. 30–5 (1983)
2   D. Benton *et al.*, 'The impact of the supply of glucose to the brain on mood and memory', *Nutr Rev*, vol 59(1 Pt 2), 2001, pp. S20–1
3   D. Benton *et al.*, 'Mild hypoglycaemia and questionnaire measures of aggression', *Biol Psychol*, vol 14(1–2), 1982, pp. 129–35
4   J. Yaryura-Tobias and F. Neziroglu, 'Violent behaviour, Brain dysrythmia and glucose dysfunction: A new syndrome', *J Ortho Psych*, vol 4, 1975, pp. 182–5
5   M. Bruce and M. Lader, 'Caffeine abstention and the management of anxiety disorders', *Psychol Med*, vol 19, 1989, pp. 211–14
6   W. Wendel and W. Beebe, 'Glycolytic activity in schizophrenia', in D. Hawkins and L. Pauling (eds), *Orthomol Psychiatry*, 1973
7   R. Prinz and D. Riddle, 'Associations between nutrition and behaviour in 5 year old children', *Nutr Rev*, vol 43, suppl., 1986
8   L. Christensen, 'Psychological distress and diet: Effects of sucrose and caffeine', *J Appl Nutr*, vol 40(1), 1988, pp. 44–50
9   D. Fullerton *et al.*, 'Sugar, opionoids and binge eating', *Brain Res Bull*, vol 14(6), 1985, pp. 273–80
10  L. Christensen, 'Psychological distress and diet: Effects of sucrose and caffeine', *J Applied Nutr*, vol 40, 1988, pp. 44–50
11  M. Colgan and L. Colgan, 'Do nutrient supplements and dietary changes affect learning and emotional reactions of children with learning difficulties? A controlled series of 16 cases', *Nutr Health*, vol 3, 1984, pp. 69–77
12  S. Schoenthaler *et al.*, 'The impact of low food additive and sucrose diet on academic performance in 803 New York City public schools', *Int J Biosocial Research*, vol 8(2), 1986, pp. 185–95
13  R. J. Prinz *et al.*, 'Dietary correlates of hyperactive behaviour in children', *J Consulting Clin Psychol*, vol 48, 1980, pp. 760–9
14  S. J. Schoenthaler *et al.*, 'The effect of randomised vitamin-mineral supplementation on violent and non-violent antisocial behaviour among incarcerated juveniles', *J Nut Env Med*, vol 7, 1997, pp. 343–52
15  L. Langseth and J. Dowd, 'Glucose tolerance and hyperkinesis', *Fd Cosmet Toxicol*, vol 16, 1978, p. 129

16 K. B. Scribner *et al.*, 'Hepatic steatosis and increased adiposity in mice consuming rapidly vs. slowly absorbed carbohydrate' *Obesity* (Silver Spring). vol 15(9), 2007, pp. 2190–9

17 R. G. Walton *et al.*, 'Adverse reactions to aspartame: Double blind challenge in patients from a vulnerable population', *J Biol Psychiatry*, vol 34(1–2), 1993, pp.13–17

18 S. E. Swithers and T. L. Davidson, 'A Role for Sweet Taste: Calorie Predictive Relations in Energy Regulation by Rats', *Behavioral Neuroscience*, vol 122(1), 2008, pp. 161–173

19 K. A. Wesnes *et al.*, 'Breakfast reduces declines in attention and memory over the morning in schoolchildren', *Appetite*, vol 41, 2003, pp. 329–31

20 K. Gilliland and D. Andress, 'Ad lib caffeine consumption, symptoms of caffeinism, and academic performance', *Am J Psychiatry*, vol 138(4), 1981, pp. 512–14

21 N. J. Richardson *et al.*, 'Mood and performance effects of caffeine in relation to acute and chronic caffeine deprivation', *Pharmacology, Biochemistry and Behavior*, vol 52(2), 1995, pp. 313–20

## Chapter 3: Fats – the good, the bad and the ugly

1 M. Makrides, 'Are long-chain polyunsaturated fatty acids essential nutrients in infancy?' *Lancet*, vol 345, 1995, pp. 1463–8

2 L. Stevens, 'Essential fat metabolism in boys with attention-deficit hyperactivity disorder', *Am J Clin Nutr*, vol 62, 1995, pp. 761–8

3 P. Willatts *et al.* 'Effect of long-chain polyunsaturated fatty acids in infant formula on problem solving at 10 months of age', *Lancet*, vol 352, 1998, pp. 688–91

4 J. B. Helland *et al.*, 'Maternal supplementation with very-long-chain n-3 fatty acids during pregnancy and lactation augments children's IQ at 4 years of age', *Pediatrics*, vol 111, 2003, pp. 39–44

5 A. J. Richardson and B. Puri, 'A randomized double-blind, placebo-controlled study of the effects of supplementation with highly unsaturated fatty acids on ADHD-related symptoms in children with specific learning difficulties', *Prog Neuropsychopharm Biol Psychiat*, vol 26(2), 2002, pp. 233–9

6 A. J. Richardson and P. Montgomery, 'The Oxford-Durham study: A randomized controlled trial of dietary supplementation with fatty acids in children with developmental coordination disorder', *Pediatrics*, vol 115, 2005, pp. 1360–6

7 L. J. Stevens *et al.*, 'Essential fat metabolism in boys with attention-deficit hyperactivity disorder', *Am J Clin Nutr*, vol 65, 1995, pp. 761–8

8 J. R. Burgess, *ADHD: observational and interventional studies*, NIH workshop on omega-3 EFAs in psychiatric disorders, National Institutes of Health, Bethesda, Maryland, US, 1988

9 A. J. Richardson and B. Puri, 'A randomized double-blind, placebo-controlled study of the effects of supplementation with highly unsaturated fatty acids on ADHD-related symptoms in children with specific learning difficulties', *Prog Neuropsychopharmacol Biol Psychiatry*, vol 26(2), 2002, pp. 233–9

10 R. DeCaterina and G. Basta, 'n-3 Fatty acids and the inflammatory response – biological background', *European Heart Journal Supplements 3*, June, 2001, Suppl D: D42–D49.

11 I. Hwang *et al.*, 'N-3 polyunsaturated fatty acids and atopy in Korean preschoolers', *Lipids*, vol 42(4) 2007, pp. 345–9

12 S. E. Carlson *et al.*, 'Long-term feeding of formulas high in linolenic acid and marine oil to very low birth weight infants: Phospholipids fatty acids', *Pediatr Res*, vol 30, 1991, pp. 404–12

13 A. J. Richardson and P. Montgomery, 'The Oxford-Durham study', *Pediatrics*, 2005

## Chapter 4: Protein power

1 W. Poldinger et al., 'A functional-dimensional approach to depression: Serotonin deficiency and target syndrome in a comparison of 5-hydroxytryptophan and fluvoxamine', *Psychopathol*, vol 24(2), 1991, pp. 53–81

2 J. B. Deijen et al., 'Tyrosine improves cognitive performance and reduces blood pressure in cadets', *Brain Research Bulletin*, vol 48(2), 1999, pp. 203–9

3 I. S. Shiah and N. Yatham, 'GABA functions in mood disorders: An update and critical review', *Nature Life Sciences*, vol 63(15) 1998, pp. 1289–1303

## Chapter 5: Vital vitamins and magic minerals

1 A. Lucas et al., 'Randomised trial of early diet in preterm babies and later intelligence quotient', *BMJ*, vol 317, 1998, pp. 1481–7

## Chapter 6: Anti-nutrients and how to avoid them

1 H. L. Needleman et al., 'The long-term effects of exposure to low doses of lead in childhood: An 11-year follow-up report', *N Engl J Med*, vol 332, 1990, pp. 83–8

2 S. Davies, editorial, *J Nut Med*, vol 2(3), 1991, pp. 227–47

3 B. Bateman et al., 'The effects of a double blind, placebo controlled, artificial food colourings and benzoate preservative challenge on hyperactivity in a general population sample of preschool children', *Archives of Disease in Childhood*, vol 89, 2004, pp. 506–511

4 D. McCann et al., 'Food additives and hyperactive behaviour in 3-year-old and 8/9-year-old children in the community: a randomised, double-blinded, placebo-controlled trial', *Lancet*, vol, 370(9598), 2007, pp. 1560–7

5 N. I. Ward et al., 'The influence of the chemical additive tartrazine on the zinc status of hyperactive children – a double-blind placebo controlled study', *J Nutr Med*, vol 1, 1990, pp. 51–7

## Chapter 7: Getting to the gut of the matter

1 L. V. Hooper et al., 'How host-microbial interactions shape the nutrient environment of the mammalian intestine', *Annu Rev Nutr*, vol 22, 2002, p. 283

## Chapter 8: Feeding your child's brain

1 B. Gesch, 'Influence of supplementary vitamins, minerals and essential fats on the antisocial behaviour of young adult prisoners', *Brit J Psychiatry*, vol 181, 2002, pp. 22–8

2 A. J. Richardson and P. Montgomery, 'The Oxford-Durham study: A randomized controlled trial of dietary supplementation with fatty acids in children with developmental coordination disorder', *Pediatrics*, vol 115, 2005, pp. 1360–6

3 A. Borjel et al., *Homocysteine Metabolism*, 5th International Conference Abstract, Italy, June 2005

4 C. M. Carter et al., 'Effects of a few food diet in attention deficit disorder', *Archives of Disease in Childhood*, vol 69, 1993, pp. 564–8

5 World Health Organization, *The World Health Report 2001 – Mental Health: New Understanding, New Hope*, WHO, 2001. Available at www.who.int/whr/2001/

6 A. Borjel et al., 'Plasma homocysteine levels, MTHFR polymorphisms 677C>T, 1298A>C, 1793G>A, and school achievement in a population sample of Swedish children', paper presented at Homocysteine Metabolism, 5th International Conference, Milano (Italy), 26–30 June, 2005

7  J. Penland, Experimental Biology conference, San Diego, 4 April, 2005 (pending publication)

## Chapter 9: Thinking faster, boosting IQ

1  A. L. Kubala and M. M. Katz, 'Nutritional factors in psychological test behaviour', *J Genet Psychol*, vol 96, 1960, pp. 343–52

2  R. F. Harrell *et al.*, Can nutritional supplements help mentally retarded children? An exploratory study. *Proc Natl Acad Sci U S A* Jan 1981, 78(1):574–8

3  D. Benton and G. Roberts, 'Effect of vitamin and mineral supplementation on intelligence of school children', *Lancet*, 1988

4  S. J. Schoenthaler *et al.*, 'Controlled trial of vitamin-mineral supplementation: Effects on intelligence and performance', *Person Individ Diff*, vol 12(4), 1991, pp. 351–2

5  Benton, D., 'Micro-nutrient supplementation and the intelligence of children', *Neurosci Biobehav* Rev, vol 25(4), 2001, pp. 297–309

6  Nemo Study Group, 'Effect of a 12-mo micronutrient intervention on learning and memory in well-nourished and marginally nourished school-aged children: Two parallel, randomized, placebo-controlled studies in Australia and Indonesia', *Am J Clin Nutr*, vol 86, 2007, pp. 1082–93

7  L. J. Whalley *et al.*, 'Cognitive aging, childhood intelligence, and the use of food supplements: Possible involvement of n-3 fatty acids', *Am J Clin Nutr*, vol 80(6), 2004, pp. 1650–7

8  W. Snowden, 'Evidence from an analysis of 2000 errors and omissions made in IQ tests by a small sample of schoolchildren, undergoing vitamin and mineral supplementation, that speed of processing is an important factor in IQ performance', *Personality & Individual Differences*, vol 22(1), Jan 1997, 131–4.

9  J. Penland, Zinc affects cognition and psychosocial function of middle-school children, Experimental Biology conference, San Diego, 4 April, 2005 (pending publication)

10  D. Benton *et al.*, 'Thiamine supplementation mood and cognitive functioning', *Psychopharmacol* (Berl), vol 129(1), 1997, pp. 66–71

11  P. Willatts *et al.*, 'Effect of long-chain polyunsaturated fatty acids in infant formula on problem solving at 10 months of age', *Lancet* , vol 352(9129), 1998, pp. 688–91

12  C. Agostoni *et al.*, 'Developmental quotient at 24 months and fatty acid composition of diet in early infancy: A follow up study', *Arch Dis Child*, vol 76(5), 1997, pp. 421–4

13  Jensen *et al.*, 'Effects of maternal docosahexaenoic acid intake on visual function and neurodevelopment in breast-fed term infants', *Am J Clin Nutr*, vol 82(1), 2005, pp. 125–32

14  I. B. Helland *et al.*, 'Maternal Supplementation With Very-Long-Chain n-3 Fatty Acids During Pregnancy and Lactation Augments Children's IQ at 4 Years of Age', *Pediatrics*, vol. 111(1), 2003, pp. e39–e44

15  E. C. Bakker *et al.*, 'Relationship between long-chain polyunsaturated fatty acids at birth and motor function at 7 years of age', *Eur J Clin Nutr*, 19 Dec., 2007 (Epub)

16  L. Horwood and D.M. Fergusson, 'Breast-feeding and later cognitive and academic outcomes', *Pediatrics*, vol 101, 1998, pp. 1–13

17  C. Lanting *et al.*, 'Neurological differences between 9-year-old children fed breast-milk or formula-milk as babies' *Lancet*, vol 344(13), 1994, pp. 9–22

## Chapter 10: Developing concentration and a sharp memory

1  D. Benton *et al.*, 'Mild hypoglycaemia and questionnaire measures of aggression', *Biol Psychol*, vol 14(1–2), 1982, pp. 129–35

2 S. Schoenthaler *et al.*, 'The impact of a low food additive and sucrose diet on academic performance in 803 New York City public schools', *Int J Biosocial Res*, vol 8(2), 1986, pp. 185–95

3 C. C. Ani and S. M. Grantham-McGregor, 'The effects of breakfast on children's educational performance, attendance and classroom behaviour', in N. Donovan and C. Street (eds), *Fit for School: How breakfast clubs meet health, education and childcare needs*, New Policy Institute, 1999, pp. 14–22, and J. L. Brown, 'New findings about child nutrition and cognitive development', in the same publication, pp. 36–44; and C. Michaud *et al.*, 'Effects of breakfast-size on short-term memory, concentration, mood and blood glucose', *Journal of Adolescent Health*, vol 12, 1991, pp. 53–7

4 D. Benton *et al.*, 'The impact of long-term vitamin supplementation on cognitive functioning', *Psychopharmacol* (Berl), vol 117(3), 1995, pp. 298–305

5 D. Benton *et al.*, 'Thiamine supplementation, mood and cognitive functioning', *Psychopharmacol* (Berl), vol 129(1), 1997, pp. 66–71

6 J. P. Jones, H. S. Swartzwelder *et al.*, 'Choline availability to the developing rat fetus alters adult hippocampal long-term potentiation', *Brain Res Dev Brain Res*, vol 118(1–2), 1999, pp. 159–67

7 S. L. Ladd *et al.*, 'Effect of phosphatidylcholine on explicit memory', *Clin Neuropharmacol*, vol 16(6), 1993, pp. 540–9

8 J. Shabert *et al.*, *The Ultimate Nutrient – Glutamine*, Avery Publications, 1990

9 T. Ziegler *et al.*, 'Safety and metabolic effects of L-glutamine administration in humans', *J Parenter Enteral Nutr*, vol 14(4 supp), 1990, pp. 137S–146S

## Chapter 11: Revving up reading and writing

1 A. J. Richardson and J. Wilmer, 'Association between fatty acid symptoms and dyslexic and ADHD characteristics in normal college students', paper given at British Dyslexia Association International Conference, University of York, April 2001

2 M. H. Jorgensen *et al.*, 'Is there a relation between docosahexaenoic acid concentration in mothers' milk and visual development in term infants?' *J Pediatr Gastroenterol Nutr*, vol 32, 2001, pp. 293–6

3 A. J. Richardson *et al.*, 'Fatty acid deficiency signs predict the severity of reading and related problems in dyslexic children', paper given at British Dyslexia Association International Conference, 2001

4 C. M. Absolon *et al.*, 'Psychological disturbance in atopic eczema: The extent of the problem in school-aged children', *Br J Dermatol*, vol 137(2), 1997, pp. 241–5

5 A. J. Richardson *et al.*, 'Abnormal cerebral phospholipid metabolism in dyslexia indicated by phosphorus-31 magnetic resonance spectroscopy', *NMR Biomed*, vol 10, 1997, pp. 309–14

6 B. J. Stordy, 'Dyslexia, attention deficit hyperactivity disorder, dyspraxia – do fatty acids help?', *Dyslexia Review*, vol 9(2), 1997, pp.1–3

7 B. J. Stordy, 'Benefit of docosahexanoic acid supplements to dark adaptation in dyslexia', *Lancet*, vol 346, 1995, p. 385

8 P. K. Hardman *et al.*, 'The effects of diet and sublingual provocative testing on eye movements with dyslexic individuals', *J Am Optom Assoc*, vol 60(1), 1989, pp. 10–13.

## Chapter 12: Obesity and being overweight

1 C. M. Boney *et al.*, 'Metabolic syndrome in childhood: association with birth weight, maternal obesity, and gestational diabetes mellitus', *Pediatrics*, vol 115(3), 2005, pp. 290–6.

2 M. W. Gillman *et al.*, 'Risk of overweight among adolescents who were breast-fed as infants', *JAMA*, vol 285(19), 2001, pp. 2461–7

3 J. C. Lumeng *et al.*, 'Shorter sleep duration is associated with increased risk for being over-weight at ages 9 to 12 years', *Pediatrics*, vol 120(5), 2007, pp. 1020–9

## Chapter 13: Protecting your child from food allergies

1 E. Young *et al.*, 'A population study of food intolerance', *Lancet*, vol 343, 1994, pp. 1127–9

2 British Society for Allergy and Environmental Medicine, *Effective Allergy Practice*, 1984

3 T. Randolph, 'Allergy as a causative factor of fatigue, irritability and behaviour problems of children', *J Pediatr*, vol 31, 1987, p. 560

4 T. Tuormaa, *An Alternative to Psychiatry*, The Book Guild, 1991

5 J. Egger *et al.*, 'Controlled trial of oligoantigenic treatment in the hyperkinetic syndrome', *Lancet*, 9 March 1985, pp. 540–5

6 J. Egger *et al.*, 'Is migraine a food allergy? A double-blind controlled trial of oligoantigenic diet treatment', *Lancet*, 15 October 1983, pp. 865–9

## Chapter 14: Sniffles, wheezes, coughs and colds

1 S. Mohammed and S. Goodacre, 'Intravenous and nebulised magnesium sulphate for acute asthma: systematic review and meta-analysis', *Emerg Med J.* vol 24(12), 2007, pp. 823–30

2 Y. Hashimoto *et al.*, 'Assessment of magnesium status in patients with bronchial asthma', *J Asthma*. 2000 vol 37(6), 2000, pp. 489–96

3 F. D. Gilliland *et al.*, 'Dietary magnesium, potassium, sodium, and children's lung func-tion', *Am J Epidemiol*, vol 155(2), 2002, pp. 125–31

4 F. D. Gilliland *et al.*, 'Children's lung function and antioxidant vitamin, fruit, juice, and vegetable intake', *Am J Epidemiol*, 2003 vol 158(6), 2003, pp. 576–84

5 T. Antova *et al.*, 'Nutrition and respiratory health in children in six Central and Eastern European countries', *Thorax*. 2003 vol 58(3), 2003, pp. 231–6

6 J. S. Burns *et al.*, 'Low dietary nutrient intakes and respiratory health in adolescents', *Chest*, 2007 vol 132(1), 2007, pp. 238–45

7 J. McCreanor *et al.*, 'Respiratory effects of exposure to diesel traffic in persons with asthma', *N Engl J Med.*, vol 357(23), 2007, pp. 2348–58

8 M. Joshua *et al.*, 'Over the Counter but No Longer under the Radar — Pediatric Cough and Cold Medications', NEJM, vol 357, 2007, pp. 2321–4

9 I. M. Paul *et al.*, 'Effect of Honey, Dextromethorphan, and No Treatment on Nocturnal Cough and Sleep Quality for Coughing Children and Their Parents', *Arch Pediatr Adolesc Med* vol 161(12), 2007, pp. 1140–6

10 I. Petersen I *et al.*, 'Protective effect of antibiotics against serious complications of common respiratory tract infections: retrospective cohort study with the UK General Practice Research Database', *BMJ*, 2007 vol 335(7627), 2007, p. 982

## Chapter 16: Overcoming eating disorders

1 K. Hambidge and A. Silverman, 'Pica with rapid improvement after dietary zinc supple-mentation', *Arch Dis Child*, vol 48, 1973, p. 567

2 D. Horrobin and S. C. Cunnane, 'Interactions between zinc, essential fatty acids and prostaglandins: Relevance to acrodermatitis enteropatica, total parenteral nutrition, and

glucagonoma syndrome, diabetes, anorexia nervosa, and sickle cell anemia', *Medical Hypothesis*, vol 6, 1980, pp. 277–96

3 R. C. Casper and A. S. Prasad, 1980, later confirmed by L. Humphries *et al.*, 'Zinc deficiency and eating disorders', *J Clin Psychiatry*, vol 50(12), 1980, pp. 456–9

4 P. R. Flanagan, 'A model to produce pure zinc deficiency in rats and its use to demonstrate that dietary phytate increases the excretion of endogenous zinc', *J Nutr*, vol 114, 1984, pp. 493–502 and A. Grider *et al.*, 'Age-dependent influence of dietary zinc restriction on short-term memory in male rats', *Physiology and Behaviour*, vol 72(3), 2001, pp. 339–48

5 A. Arcasoy *et al.*, 'Ultrastructural changes in the mucosa of the small intestine in patients with geophagia (Prasad's syndrome)', *J Pediatr Gastroenterol Nutr*, vol 11(2), 1990, pp. 279–82

6 D. Bryce-Smith and R. I. Simpson, 'Case of anorexia nervosa responding to zinc sulphate', *Lancet*, vol 2(8398), 1984, p. 350

7 Katz *et al.*, 'Zinc deficiency in anorexia nervosa', *J Adol Health Care*, vol 8, 1987, pp. 400–6

8 L. Humphries *et al.*, 'Zinc deficiency and eating disorders', *J Clin Psychiatry*, 1989

9 N. F. Shay and H. F. Mangian HF, 'Neurobiology of zinc-influenced eating behavior', *J Nutr*, vol 130(5S Suppl), 2000, pp. 1493S–9S

10 R. Bakan *et al.*, 'Dietary zinc intake of vegetarian and non-vegetarian patients with anorexia nervosa', *Int J Eat Disord*, vol 13(2), 1993, pp. 229–33

11 F. Askenazy *et al.*, 'Whole blood serotonin content, tryptophan concentrations, and impulsivity in anorexia nervosa', *Biological Psychiatry*, vol 43(3), 1998, pp. 188–95

12 A. Favaro, 'Tryptophan levels, excessive exercise, and nutritional status in anorexia nervosa', *Psychosomatic Medicine*, vol 62(4), 2000, pp. 535–8

13 P. J. Cowen and K. A. Smith, 'Serotonin, dieting, and bulimia nervosa', *Advances in Experimental Medicine and Biology*, vol 467, 1999, pp. 101–4

## Chapter 17: Curing sleep problems

1 Y. Harrison and J. A. Horne, 'Sleep deprivation affects speech', *Sleep*, vol 20(10), 1997, pp. 871–7

2 L. Ozturk *et al.*, 'Effects of 48 hours sleep deprivation on human immune profile', *Sleep Res Online*, vol 2(4), 1999, pp. 107–11

3 M. G. Smits *et al.* 'Melatonin for chronic sleep onset insomnia in children: A randomized placebo-controlled trial', *J Child Neurol*, vol 16(2), 2001, pp. 86–92

4 E. J. Pavonen *et al.* 'Effectiveness of melatonin in the treatment of sleep disturbances in children with Asperger disorder', *J Child Adolesc Psychopharmacol*, vol 13(1), 2003, pp. 83–95

## Chapter 18: Enhancing mood and behaviour

1 J. R. Hibbeln, 'Fish consumption and major depression', *Lancet*, vol 351, 1998, pp. 1213

2 B. Nemets *et al.*, 'Addition of omega-3 fatty acid to maintenance medication treatment for recurrent unipolar depressive disorder', *American Journal of Psychiatry*, vol 159, 2002, pp. 477–9; L. Marangell *et al.*, 'A Double-Blind, Placebo-Controlled Study of the Omega-3 Fatty Acid Docosahexaenoic Acid (DHA) in the Treatment of Major Depression', *American Journal of Psychiatry*, vol 160, 2003, pp. 996–8; A. L. Stoll *et al.*, 'Omega 3 Fatty Acids in Bipolar Disorder: A Preliminary Double-Blind, Placebo-Controlled Trial,' *Archives of General Psychiatry*, vol 56, 1999, pp. 407–12; M. R. Smith, *et al.*, 'Fatty Acid Composition in Major Depression: Decreased w3 Fractions in Cholesteryl Esters And Increased C20:4 Omega 6/C20:5 Omega 3 Ratio in Cholesteryl Esters and Phospholipids', *Journal of Affective Disorders*, vol 38, 1996, pp. 35–46; M. Peet *et al.*, 'Depletion of Omega-3 Fatty Acid

Levels in Red Blood Cell Membranes of Depressive Patient', *Biological Psychiatry* vol 43, 1998, pp. 315–19

3  B. Puri *et al.*, 'Eicosapentaenoic acid in treatment-resistant depression', *Archives of General Psychiatry*, vol 59(1), 2002, Letters to the Editor

4  J. A. Blumenthal *et al.*, 'Exercise and pharmacotherapy in the treatment of major depressive disorder', *Psychosom Med*, vol 69(7), 2007, 587–96

5  K. A. Smith *et al.*, 'Relapse of depression after rapid depletion of tryptophan', *Lancet*, vol 349, 1997, pp. 915–19

6  E. H. Turner *et al.*, 'Serotoninalacarte: Supplementation with the serotonin precursor 5-hydroxytryptophan', *Pharmacology and Therapeutics* vol 109(3), 2006, pp. 325–38

7  H. Cass, 'SAMe – the master tuner supplement for the 21st century', published on www.naturallyhigh.co.uk, 2001

8  P. G. Janicak *et al.*, 'Parenteral S-adenosyl-methionine (SAMe) in depression: Literature review and preliminary data', *Psychopharmacol Bull*, vol 25(2), 1989, pp. 238–42

9  T. Hamazaki *et al.*, 'The effect of docosahexaenoic acid on aggression in young adults: A placebo-controlled double-blind study', *J Clin Invest*, vol 97, 1996, pp. 1129–33

10  S. J. Schoenthaler *et al.*, 'The effect of randomised vitamin-mineral supplementation on violent and non-violent antisocial behaviour among incarcerated juveniles', *J Nut Env Med*, vol 7, 1997, pp. 343–52

11  J. Egger *et al.*, 'Controlled trial of oligoantigenic treatment in the hyperkinetic syndrome', *Lancet*, vol 1(8428), 1985, pp. 540–5

12  A. G. Schauss and C. E. Simonsen, 'A critical analysis of the diets of chronic juvenile offenders', Part 1, *J Orthomol Psychiatry*, vol. 8(3), 1979, pp. 149–57

13  D. Papalos and J. Papalos, *The Bipolar Child*, Broadway Books, 2000

## Chapter 19: Drug-free solutions for ADHD

1  A. Richardson, 'Fatty acids in dyslexia, dyspraxia, ADHD and the autistic spectrum', *The Nutrition Practitioner*, vol 3(3), 2001, pp. 18–24

2  R. J. Prinz *et al.*, 'Dietary correlates of hyperactive behaviour in children, *J Consulting Clin Psychol*, vol 48, 1980, pp. 760–9

3  S. J. Schoenthaler *et al.*, 'The effect of randomised vitamin-mineral supplementation on violent and non-violent antisocial behaviour among incarcerated juveniles', *J Nut Env Med*, 1997

4  L. Langseth and J. Dowd, 'Glucose tolerance and hyperkinesis', *Fd Cosmet Toxicol*, vol 16, 1978, p. 129

5  I. Colquhon and S. Bunday, 'A lack of essential fats as a possible cause of hyperactivity in children', *Medical Hypotheses*, vol 7, 1981, pp. 673–9

6  L. J. Stevens *et al.*, 'Essential fat metabolism in boys with attention-deficit hyperactivity disorder', *Am J Clin Nutr*, vol 65, 1995, pp. 761–8

7  J. R. Burgess, *ADHD: observational and interventional studies*, NIH workshop on omega-3 EFAs in psychiatric disorder, National Institutes of Health, Bethesda, Maryland, 1998

8  A. J. Richardson and B. Puri, 'A randomized double-blind, placebo-controlled study of the effects of supplementation with highly unsaturated fatty acids on ADHD-related symptoms in children with specific learning difficulties', *Prog Neuropsychopharmacol Biol Psychiatry*, vol 26(2), 2002, pp. 233–9

9  A. Richardson and B. Puri, 'A randomized double-blind, placebo-controlled study of the effects of supplementation with highly unsaturated fatty acids on ADHD, *Prog Neuropsychopharmacol Biol Psychiatry*, 2002

10  B. O'Reilly, Hyperactive Children's Support Group Conference, London, June 2001

11  M. D. Boris and F. S. Mandel, 'Foods and additives are common causes of the attention deficit hyperactive disorder in children', *Ann Allergy*, vol. 72 (1994), pp. 462–8

12  R. J. Theil, 'Nutrition based interventions for ADD and ADHD', *Townsend Letter for Doctors & Patients*, April 2000, pp. 93–5

13  A. R. Swain *et al.*, 'Salicylates, oligoantigenic diet and behaviour', *Lancet*, vol. 2(8445), 1985, pp. 41–2

14  B. Starobrat-Hermelin and T. Kozielec, 'The effects of magnesium physiological supplementation on hyperactivity in children with attention deficit hyperactivity disorder (ADHD): Positive response to magnesium oral loading test', *Magnes Res*, vol 10(2), 1997, pp. 149–56

15  N. I. Ward, 'Assessment of clinical factors in relation to child hyperactivity', *J Nutr Environ Med*, vol 7, 1997, pp. 333–42

16  N. I. Ward, 'Hyperactivity and a previous history of antibiotic usage', *Nutrition Practitioner*, vol 3(3), 2001, p. 12

17  N. D. Volkow *et al.*, 'Therapeutic doses of oral methylphenidate significantly increase extracellular dopamine in the human brain', *J Neuroscience*, vol 21(RC121), 2001, pp. 1–5

18  S. Chaplin, *The Prescriber*, 5 August 2005, www.escriber.com

19  Dr Joan Baizer of the State University of New York at Buffalo at the Annual Meeting of the Society for Neuroscience, 11 November 2001

20  See www.blockcenter.com/articles2/ritalin_dea.htm and R. D. Ciaranello, 'Attention deficit-hyperactivity disorder and resistance to thyroid hormone – a new idea?', *N Engl J Med*, vol 328(14), 1993, pp. 1038–9

21  National Institutes of Health, *NIH Consensus Statement: Diagnosis and Treatment of Attention Deficit Hyperactivity Disorder (ADHD)*, NIH, 1998

22  N. Lambert and C. Hartsough, 'Prospective study of tobacco smoking and substance dependencies among samples of ADHD and non-ADHD participants,' *Journal of Learning Disabilities*, vol 31, 1998, pp. 533–44

23  See the Optimal Wellness Centre website www.mercola.com/2001/jan/7/lendon_smith.htm, and www.smithsez.com/ADHDandADD.html

## Chapter 20: Moving off the autistic spectrum

1  R. Huff, *US State Department of Developmental Services Report on Autism*, 1999

2  B. Rimland *et al.*, 'The effect of high doses of vitamin B6 on autistic children: A double-blind crossover study', *Am J Psychiatry*, vol 135(4), 1978, pp. 472–5

3  S. I. Pfeiffer *et al.*, 'Efficacy of vitamin B6 and magnesium in the treatment of autism: A methodology review and summary of outcomes', *J Autism Dev Disord*, vol 25(5), p1995, pp. 481–93

4  J. Martineau *et al.*, 'Vitamin B6, magnesium, and combined B6-Mg: Therapeutic effects in childhood autism', *Biol Psychiatry*, vol 20(5), 1985, pp. 467–78

5  S. Vancassel *et al.*, 'Plasma fatty acid levels in autistic children', *Prostaglandins Leukot Essent Fatty Acids*, vol 65, 2001, pp. 1–7

6  J. G. Bell *et al.*, 'Red blood cell fatty acid compositions in a patient with autism spectrum disorder: a characteristic abnormality in neurodevelopmental disorders?', *Prostaglandins Leukot Essent Fatty Acids*, vol 63(1–2), 2000, pp. 21–5

7  J. G. Bell, 'Fatty acid deficiency and phospholipase A2 in autistic spectrum disorders', workshop report, St Anne's College, Oxford, September 2001

8  M. Megson, 'Is autism a G-Alpha protein defect reversible with natural vitamin A?', *Medical Hypotheses*, vol 54(6), 2000, pp. 979–83

9 M. Megson, *The biological basis for perceptual deficits in autism: Vitamin A and G-proteins*, lecture given at Ninth International Symposium on Functional Medicine, May 2002

10 Paul Whiteley, the Sunderland University Autism Unit, 'The Biology of Autism – Unravelled' presentation given at the Autism Unravelled Conference, London, May 2001

11 Paul Whitely *et al.*, 'A gluten free diet as an intervention for autism and associated disorders: Preliminary findings', *Autism: International J of Research and Practice*, vol 3, 1999, pp. 45–65

12 'Anti-fungal drugs more helpful than Ritalin in autistic children', Letter to the Editor, *Townsend Letter for Doctors and Patients*, April 2001, p. 99

13 A. J. Wakefield *et al.*, 'Enterocolitis in children with developmental disorders', *Am J Gastroenterol*, vol 95(9), 2000, pp. 2285–95

14 M. A. Brudnak, 'Application of genomeceuticals to the molecular and immunological aspects of autism', *Medical Hypotheses*, vol 57(2), 2001, pp. 186–91

15 P. Varmanen *et al.*, 'S54X-prolyl dipeptidyl aminopeptidase gene (pepX) is part of the glnRA operon in *Lactobaccilus rhamnosus*', *J Bacteriol*, vol 182(1), 2000, pp. 146–54

16 Paul Whitely *et al.*, 'A gluten free diet as an intervention for autism and associated disorders: Preliminary findings', *Autism: International J of Research and Practice*, 1999

17 J. Robert Cade, University of Florida Department of Medicine and Physiology, at www.panix.com/~paleodiet/autism/cadelet.txt

18 M. Ash and E. Gilmore, 'Modifying autism through functional nutrition', paper given at Allergy Research Group conference, London, January 2001

19 Dr Rosemary Waring, University of Birmingham School of Biosciences, 'Sulphate, sulphation and gut permeability: are cytokines involved?' Autism Unravelled Conference Proceedings, London, 11 May, 2001

20 A. J. Wakefield *et al.*, 'Ileal-lymphoid hyperplasia, non-specific colitis, and pervasive developmental disorder in children', *Lancet*, vol 351, 1998, pp. 637–41

21 A. J. Wakefield, speaking at the Allergy Research Foundation conference, November 1999

22 F. E. Yazbak, 'Autism – is there a vaccine connection?', see www.autisme.net/Yazbak1.htm

23 B. Rimland, *J Nut Env Med*, vol 10, 2000, pp. 267–9

24 Ibid. See also Ashcraft & Gerel (law firm), 'Autism caused by childhood vaccinations containing Thimerosal or mercury', at www.ashcraftandgerel.com/thimerosal. html

25 B. Rimland, 'Parents' ratings of the effectiveness of drugs and nutrients', *Autism Research Review International*, vol 8, October 1994

26 D. B. Smith and E. Obbens, 'Antifolate-antiepileptic relationships', in M. I. Botez and E. H. Reynolds, eds, *Folic Acid in Neurology, Psychiatry and Internal Medicine*, Raven Press, 1979

27 F. B. Gibberd *et al.*, 'The influence of folic acid on the frequency of epileptic attacks', *Europ J Clin Pharmacology*, vol 19(1), 1981, pp. 57–60

28 D. B. Smith and E. Obbens, 'Antifolate-antiepileptic relationships', in M. I. Botez and E. H. Reynolds, eds, *Folic Acid in Neurology, Psychiatry and Internal Medicine*, Raven Press, 1979

29 M. Nakazawa, 'High dose vitamin B6 therapy in infantile spasms – the effect of adverse reactions', *Brain and Development*, vol 5(2), 1983, p. 193

30 J. Pietz *et al.*, 'Treatment of infantile spasms with high-dosage vitamin B6', *Epilepsia*, vol 34(4), 1993, pp. 757–63

31 A. Sohler and C. Pfeiffer, 'A direct method for the determination of managanese in whole blood: patients with seizure activity have low blood levels', *J Orthomol Psychiat*, vol 12, 1983, pp. 215–34

32 P. S. Papavasiliou *et al.*, 'Seizure disorders and trace metals: Manganese tissue levels in treated epileptics', *Neurology*, vol 29, 1979, p. 1466

33 Y. Tanaka, 'Low manganese level may trigger epilepsy', *JAMA*, vol 238, 1977, p. 1805

34 C. Pfeiffer *et al.*, 'Zinc and manganese in the schizophrenias', *J Orthomol Psychiat*, vol 12, 1983, pp. 215–34

35 Y. Shoji, 'Serum magnesium and zinc in epileptic children', *Brain and Development*, vol 5(2), 1983, p. 200

36 S. K. Gupta *et al.*, 'Serum magnesium levels in idiopathic epilepsy', *J Assoc Physicians India*, vol 42(6), 1994, pp. 456–7

37 L. F. Gorges *et al.*, 'Effect of magnesium on epileptic foci', *Epilepsia*, vol 19(1), 1978, pp. 81–91

38 C. L. Zhang *et al.*, 'Paroxysmal epileptiform discharges in temporal lobe slices after prolonged exposure to low magnesium are resistant to clinically used anticonvulsants', *Epilepsy Res*, vol 20(2), 1995, pp. 105–11

39 Y. Shoji, 'Serum magnesium and zinc in epileptic children', *J Orthomol Psychiat*, 1983

40 A. Barbeau *et al.*, 'Zinc, taurine and epilepsy', *Arch Neurol*, vol 30, 1974, pp. 52–8

41 M. I. Botez *et al.*, 'Thiamine and folate treatment of chronic epileptic patients: A controlled study with the Wechsler IQ scale', *Epilepsy-Res*, vol 16(2), 1993, pp. 157–63, and A. Keyser, 'Epileptic manifestations and vitamin B1 deficiency', *Eur-Neurol*, vol 31(3), 1991, pp. 121–5

42 V. T. Ramaeckers, 'Selenium deficiency triggering intractable seizures', *Neuropediatrics*, vol 25(4), 1994, pp. 217–23

43 I. R. Tupeev, 'The antioxidant system in the dynamic combined treatment of epilepsy patients with traditional anticonvulsant preparations and an antioxidant – alpha-tocopherol', *Biull Eksp Biol Med*, vol 116(10), 1993, pp. 362–4

44 C. Christiansen *et al.*, 'Anticonvulsant action of vitamin D in epileptic patients? A controlled pilot study', *Br Med J*, 2(913), 1974, pp. 258–9

45 G. H. Johnson and F. Willis, 'Seizures as the presenting feature of rickets in an infant', *Med J Aust*, 178(9), 2003, pp. 467–8

46 F. E. Ali *et al.*, 'Loss of seizure control due to anticonvulsant-induced hypocalcemia', *Ann Pharmacother*, vol 38(6), 2004, pp. 1002–5

47 S. Yehuda, 'Essential fat preparation (SR-3) raises the seizure threshold in rats', *Eur J Pharmacol*, vol 254(1–2), 1994, pp. 193–8

48 S. Schlanger, M. Shinitzky and D. Yam, 'Diet enriched with omega-3 fatty acids alleviates convulsion symptoms in epilepsy patients,' *Epilepsia*, vol 43(1), 2002, pp. 103–4

49 B. K. Puri, 'The safety of evening primrose oil in epilepsy', *Prostaglandins Leukot Essent Fatty Acids*, vol 77(2), 2007, pp. 101–3

50 E. S. Roach *et al.*, 'N,N-dimethylglycine for epilepsy', Letter to the Editor, *N Engl J Med*, vol 307, 1982, pp. 1081–2

51 R. Huxtable *et al.*, 'The prolonged anticonvulsnat action of taurine on genetically determined seizure-susceptibility', *Canadian J Neurol Sci*, vol 5, 1978, p. 220

52 D. A. Richards *et al.*, 'Extracellular GABA in the ventrolateral thalamus of rats exhibiting spontaneous absence epilepsy: A microdialysis study', *J Neurochem*, vol 65(4), 1995, pp. 1674–80

53 J. Schmidt, 'Comparative studies on the anti-convulsant effectiveness of nootropic drugs in kindled rats', *Biomed Biochim Acta*, vol 49(5), 1990, pp. 413–19

## Chapter 21: Getting off to a good start

1 'Promotion of breast-feeding', *Journal of American Dietetic Association*, no. 97, 1997, pp. 662–6

2 M. Martin, 'Is DHA the secret of breast milk's success?' *WorldNetDaily.com*, 2002

3 E. L. Mortensen *et al.*, 'The association between duration of breast-feeding and adult intelligence', *JAMA*, vol 287, 2002, pp. 2365–71

4 F. Martinez, 'Evaluation of plasma tocopherols in relation to hematological indices of Brazilian infants on human milk and cows' milk regime from birth to 1 year of age' *American Journal of Clinical Nutrition*, vol. 41(3), 1985, p. 969

5 C. Kunz, *International Journal for Vitamin & Nutrient Research*, vol. 54(141), 1984

6 W. Craig, *Nutrition Reports International*, vol 30(4), 1984, p. 1003

7 J. Armstrong, J. J. Reilly and the Child Health Information Team, 'Breast-feeding and lowering the risk of childhood obesity', *Lancet*, vol 359(9322), 2002, pp. 2003–4

8 R. L. William et al., 'Use of antibiotics in preventing recurrent acute otitis media and in treating otitis media with effusion', JAMA, vol 270, 1993, pp. 1344–51

9 J. Braly and R. Hoggan, *Dangerous Grains*, Avery, 2002, p. 24

## Chapter 23: Finding the end of the rainbow

1 J. C. Lumeng and T. M. Cardinal, 'Providing information about a flavor to preschoolers: effects on liking and memory for having tasted it', *Chem Senses*. 2007, 32(6), 2007, pp. 505–13

# Recommended reading

Elliot, R., *The Bean Book*, Thorsons, 2000

Cousins, B., *Cooking Without Made Easy*, Harper Thorsons, 2005

Halvorsen, R., *The Truth About Vaccines: How We Are Used As Guinea Pigs Without Knowing It*, Gibson Square, 2007

Holford, P., *The Optimum Nutrition Bible*, Piatkus, 2009

Holford, P. and Lawson, S., *Optimum Nutrition Before, During and After Pregnancy*, Piatkus, 2009

Holford, P. and Braly, J., *Hidden Food Allergies*, Piatkus, 2009

Holford, P. and McDonald Joyce, F., *The Low-GL Diet Cookbook*, Piatkus, 2010

Holford, P. and McDonald Joyce, F., *Smart Food for Smart Kids*, Piatkus, 2010

Wigmore, A., *The Sprouting Book*, Avery, 1986

# Resources

## Nutrition

**The Brain Bio Centre** is the London-based treatment clinic of the charity Food for the Brain (see below). The clinic puts the optimum nutrition approach into practice for people with mental health problems, including learning difficulties, dyslexia, ADHD, autism, Alzheimer's, dementia, memory loss, depression, anxiety and schizophrenia. Deborah Colson is a child specialist at the clinic. For more information, call 020 8332 9600 or visit www.brainbiocentre.com.

**Food for the Brain** is an educational charity that promotes the link between optimum nutrition and mental health. Patrick Holford is CEO of the charity. The Food for the Brain Child Survey compared dietary habits with behaviour and learning in over 10,000 children. You can find the full results on the charity's website. Food for the Brain also provide a free child's diet transformation pack to help you improve your child's health. For more information, visit www.foodforthebrain.org.

**The Institute for Optimum Nutrition** (ION) offers a three-year foundation degree course in nutritional therapy. It also runs a clinic, has a list of nutrition practitioners across the UK, an information service and a quarterly journal, *Optimum Nutrition*.

For more information, contact ION at Avalon House, 72 Lower Mortlake Road, Richmond TW9 2JY, call 020 8614 7800 or visit www.ion.ac.uk.

To find a recommended nutritional therapist in your area, visit www.patrickholford.com and click on 'Advice' and then 'Find a Nutritionist'.

# Support for children and parents

**ChildLine** is a free helpline for children and young people in the UK, who can talk to counsellors about any problem, 24 hours a day, 365 days a year. For more information, call 0800 1111.

**The Hyperactive Children's Support Group** (HACSG) is a UK-based charity that offers support and information to parents and professionals who wish to pursue a drug-free approach to treating ADHD. It helps and supports hyperactive children and their parents, conducts research, investigates its causes and treatments, and publishes information on the condition. There are some local groups in the UK, started by the parents of hyperactive children, and there are also contact parents who are willing to help newly joined members in their area. For more information, contact HACSG at 71 Whyke Lane, Chichester, West Sussex PO19 7PD, UK, (please enclose a SAE for all general information, articles and diet booklets), call 01243 539966 or visit www.hacsg.org.uk.

**The National Autistic Society** (UK) is a charity that aims to encourage a better understanding of autism and to pioneer specialist services for people with autism and those who care for them. For more information, contact The National Autistic Society at 393 City Road, London EC1V 1NG, call 020 7833 2299 or visit www.nas.org.uk.

**Dyslexia Action** is an educational charity for the assessment and teaching of people with dyslexia, and for the training of teachers. It can assess your child using a psychological test, although most schools also offer testing (this is necessary for extra time allowance in exams), as well as providing special needs teachers to help your child with their specific areas of difficulties. For more information, contact Dyslexia Action at Park House, Wick Road, Egham, Surrey, TW20 0HH, UK, call 01784 222300, email info@dyslexiaaction.org.uk or visit www.dyslexiaaction.org.uk.

**Beating Eating Disorders** provides help and support for people affected by eating disorders, particularly anorexia nervosa, bulimia and binge eating. Call its youthline on 0845 634 7650 or visit www.b-eat.co.uk.

# Laboratory testing

**Food allergy (IgG ELISA) and homocysteine testing** is available through YorkTest Laboratories, using a home test kit whereby you can take your own finger-prick blood sample and return it to the lab for analysis. For more information, call freephone 0800 0746185 or visit www.yorktest.com.

**Hair mineral analyses** are available from Trace Elements, Inc (US), a leading laboratory for hair mineral analysis for healthcare professionals worldwide. For more information, contact the UK agent, Mineral Check, at Bull Cottage, Lenham Heath Road, Lenham Heath, Maidstone, Kent ME17 2BP,UK, call 01622 850500 or visit www.mineralcheck.com or www.traceelements.com.

**Biolab** carries out blood tests for essential fats, urine tests for urinary HPL, chemical sensitivity panels, toxic element screens and more, but only through qualified practitioners. For more information, contact Biolab at Biolab Medical Unit, The Stone House, 9 Weymouth Street, London W1W 6DB, UK, call 020 7636 5959 or visit www.biolab.co.uk.

# Products

**Living Foods** is a seed-sprouting specialist. It has everything you need to start sprouting your own seeds, including starter kits from £6. For more information, contact Living Foods at Pier House, Quay Street, St Ives, Cornwall TR26 1PT, call 01736 791 981 or visit www.sproutingseeds.co.uk.

**Bates Method** for natural eyesight improvement. Visit www.seeing.org for information on the method and to locate a teacher.

# Supplements

## Multivitamin and mineral supplements

The best chewable multivitamin, based on optimum nutrition levels, is Biocare's Optimum Nutrition for Children. For older children who can swallow capsules, Biocare's Optimum Nutrition Formula is ideal. Calma-C from Higher Nature provides additional calcium and magnesium for growing children as a pleasant-tasting drink.

Biocare make an excellent range of liquid mineral and vitamin products. These can be added in drop form to other drinks and food.

## Essential fats and fish oil supplements

The most important omega-3 fats are DHA and EPA, the richest source being cod liver oil. The most important omega-6 fat is GLA, the richest source being borage (also known as starflower) oil. Our favourite supplement is Biocare's Essential Omegas, which provides a highly concentrated mix of EPA, DHA and GLA in an ideal ratio. Equazen's Eye Q is also good.

Seven Seas makes a very good Extra High Strength Cod Liver Oil, which also contains vitamin A. Nutri's Eskimo-3 or Eskimo for Kids are very good sources of EPA and DHA – the kids version being a non-fishy-tasting liquid, while the original is a fairly neutral unflavoured version.

Vegetarian options do not provide EPA and DHA directly, only the precursors – so they're not our first choice for these omega-3s. But if you want to go for this, choose an Omega Nutrition product from Higher Nature – either oil, flavoured oil or capsules. If you choose a flavoured oil and your child has food allergies, check the list of ingredients carefully.

## Probiotics

We recommend Higher Nature's Acidobifidus powder or Biocare's Strawberry or Banana Acidophilus, a powder to be added to food or drink. Infants need a particular age-appropriate strain of probiotic available from Biocare called Bifidobacterium Infantis. Older children who can swallow capsules can take Biocare's Bio-Acidophilus. Saccharomyces boulardii, while not strictly a probiotic, plays a very important role in improving gut immunity. It is available from Nutri.

## Homocysteine-lowering nutrients

Several companies produce good homocysteine-lowering formulations. Biocare makes Connect and Solgar has Homocysteine Modulators. Connect has the advantage of containing B12 in the form of methyl-cobalamin, which is the most effective form. Homocysteine-lowering nutrients are usually only needed for a few weeks or months at the most.

### Brain support and phospholipid supplements

Additional brain nutrients include phospholipids such as phosphatidyl choline and phosphatidyl serine, and pyroglutamate and DMAE. Phosphatidyl choline (PC) can be found in lecithin granules which are a pleasant-tasting addition to breakfast. Higher Nature's High PC Lecithin Granules contain 30 per cent more PC than other lecithins. Biocare's Brain Food Formula contains a blend of these brain support nutrients.

## Company directory

### In the UK

The following companies produce good-quality supplements that are widely available in the UK.

**Biocare** produces a wide range of nutritional and herbal supplements, including an excellent children's range, which are available in good health food shops. For your nearest supplier, call 0121 433 3727 or visit www.biocare.co.uk.

**Higher Nature** produces an extensive range of nutritional and herbal supplements, which are available in good health food shops and by mail order. For your nearest supplier, call 0800 458 4747, or email info@higher-nature.co.uk or visit www.highernature.co.uk.

**Nutri** produces a range of nutritional supplements, including child-friendly fish oils such as the Eskimo range and saccharomyces boulardii (product name Gi-Sol), which are available in good health food shops. For your nearest supplier, call 0800 212 742.

**Seven Seas** specialises in cod liver oil. Its products are available in health food shops, pharmacies and supermarkets, or visit www.sseas.com.

**Solgar** produces a wide range of nutritional and herbal supplements, which are available in good health food shops. For your nearest supplier, call 01442 890 355 or visit www.solgar.co.uk.

**Totally Nourish** is an online health food store that stocks many health products including home test kits and supplements. Visit www.totallynourish.com or call freephone 0800 085 7749.

## In other regions

**South Africa** Bioharmony produces a wide range of products in South Africa and other African countries. For details of your nearest supplier contact 021 910 2767 or visit www.bioharmony.co.za.

**Australia** Solgar supplements are available in Australia. Contact Solgar on 1800 029 871 (free call) for your nearest supplier. Website: www.solgar.com.au. Another good brand is Blackmores.

**New Zealand** Biocare products are available in New Zealand. Contact Aurora Natural Therapies, 12A Battys Road, Springlands, Blenheim 7201, New Zealand. Website: www.aurora.org.nz.

**Singapore** Biocare products are available in Singapore. Contact Essential Living on 6276 1380 for your nearest supplier or visit www.essliv.com.

# Index

Note: page numbers in **bold** refer to diagrams, page numbers in *italics* refer to information contained in tables.

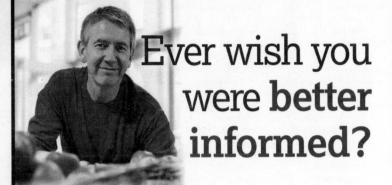

# Ever wish you were **better** informed?

**Join my 100% Health Club today and you'll receive:**

✔ My newsletter, plus Special Reports on vital health topics

✔ Immediate access to hundreds of health articles and special reports.

✔ Have your questions answered in our Members Only blogs.

✔ Save money on supplements, books and other health products.

✔ Save up to £50 on Patrick Holford's **100% Health Workshop**.

✔ Become part of a community of like-minded people and help others.

JOIN TODAY at **www.patrickholford.com**

" Being a member has transformed my life, and that of many of my family and friends. Patrick's information is always spot on and really practical. My member benefits and discounts save me much more than the subscription. Being a member is a must if you want to be and stay healthy. "

Joyce Taylor